Cocaine

DRUGS OF ABUSE
A Comprehensive Series for Clinicians

Volume 1   MARIJUANA
Mark S. Gold, M.D.

Volume 2   ALCOHOL
Norman S. Miller, M.D., and Mark S. Gold, M.D.

Volume 3   COCAINE
Mark S. Gold, M.D.

Cocaine

Mark S. Gold, M.D.

Departments of Neuroscience and Psychiatry
University of Florida College of Medicine
Gainesville, Florida

Plenum Medical Book Company
New York and London

Library of Congress Cataloging-in-Publication Data

Gold, Mark S.
    Cocaine / Mark S. Gold.
        p.   cm. -- (Drugs of abuse)
    Includes bibliographical references and index.
    ISBN 0-306-44386-4
    1. Cocaine habit. 2. Cocaine--Physiological effect. 3. Cocaine
habit--Treatment.   I. Title. II. Series: Drugs of abuse (New York,
N.Y.)
RC568.C6G653 1993
616.86'47--dc20   92-45165
                                                               CIP

ISBN 0-306-44386-4

© 1993 Plenum Publishing Corporation
233 Spring Street, New York, N.Y. 10013

Plenum Medical Book Company is an imprint of Plenum Publishing Corporation

Printed in the United States of America

Preface

For every news story in the popular press detailing the horrors and the violence associated with cocaine, there have been corresponding studies in the medical literature shedding new light on our understanding of this most troublesome drug. Our knowledge of addiction, and specifically cocaine addiction, has increased dramatically within the last few years. We stand on the threshold of an exciting new era in addictionology that promises better treatments, improved diagnostic procedures, and more effective preventative strategies. We must prepare today for the avalanche of exciting discoveries that will arrive in the coming years.

Along with the first two volumes in this series, *Marijuana* and *Alcohol*, this book strives to help the general medical community to stay abreast of the latest medical information on addiction, while presenting a fundamental resource on the neurobiology, physiology, epidemiology, history, diagnosis, treatment, and prevention of cocaine abuse. In addition, the comorbidity of cocaine abuse and eating disorders, depression, anxiety, hypertension, and various other disorders is discussed in detail. Finally, the last chapter presents new strategies tailored to specific patient groups and aimed at confronting the ever-changing face of drug abuse.

The medical community should realize that the recent and dramatic decline in drug use, detailed in Chapter 1, has stemmed primarily from educational efforts aimed at preventing drug use. This educational undertaking derived largely from the medical and research efforts that proved the deleterious effects of cocaine abuse. Clinicians, researchers, residents, and students alike must not ignore the valuable role they can play as educators in their community.

Similarly, while our gains in scientific study have been impressive, we must never lose sight of the immense task that lies ahead. Drug abuse remains a formidable problem that continues to plague our society. More addiction, younger users—the drug problem is not just going away. We must never become complacent in our knowledge of drug abuse or in our efforts to overcome this devastating disease.

Finally, I would like to thank my students and colleagues at the University of Florida, especially Allen H. Neims, M.D., Ph.D., Joel B. Cohen, Ph.D., Dwight L. Evans, M.D., and William G. Luttge, Ph.D., for their regular and critical review of my work.

MARK S. GOLD, M.D.

Contents

1

Cocaine in the 1990s

Despite significant reductions, cocaine consumption remains a formidable problem in the 1990s.

- In 1991, 6.4 million people over 12 years old used cocaine within the past year.[1]
- Among high school seniors in the class of 1991, 7.8% have used cocaine.[2]
- The cost of treating infants exposed to cocaine is estimated to be $500 million a year.[3]
- Hospital emergency room mentions of cocaine increased in the first two quarters of 1991 to 47,652 from 41,306 in 1990.[4]

In addition, there is a growing awareness among physicians of the medical and psychiatric complications of cocaine use. A 1990 report from the large-scale Epidemiologic Catchment Area Study conducted by the National Institute of Mental Health found that more than 76% of cocaine abusers also experienced anxiety disorders or depression. Cocaine-related medical complications include arrhythmias, myocardial infarctions, left ventricular hypertrophy, myocardial ischemia, coronary atherosclerosis, pneumonia, pulmonary edema, pneumothorax, pneumopericardium, seizures, impotence, gynecomastia, galactorrhea, and amenorrhea.

Furthermore, in the United States, approximately 28% of patients with acquired immunodeficiency syndrome (AIDS) are intravenous drug users who may have acquired the human immunodeficiency virus (HIV) through contaminated needles. Although the majority of these drug users abuse heroin, there has been a recent increase in intravenous cocaine use. The combination of cocaine use and AIDS poses two problems: First, evidence suggests that cocaine may suppress the human immune system and inhibit the immunological response to the opportunistic infections that may accompany HIV infection. Second, cocaine abuse can produce psychiatric and neurological symptoms such as depression, panic attacks, anorexia, arrhythmias, seizures, hallucinations, and insomnia that are also associated with AIDS. The appearance of these symptoms may impede the early identification of HIV infection.

For many years, the problems associated with cocaine abuse seemed insurmountable. The seemingly daily accounts of the addiction, violence, and destruction that accompanied the cocaine epidemic of the 1980s, combined with the much-publicized deaths of celebrities such as John Belushi and Len Bias, created an atmosphere of uncontrolled drug use that threatened American society. Fortunately, at that time a national plan designed to reduce demand *and* supply took effect. A wide range of efforts supported by schools, businesses, grass-roots organizations, medical authorities, and governmental forces united to reduce drug abuse.

Prevention: The Best Treatment

Central to the antidrug strategy was the concept that *education leads to prevention* and that ultimately prevention is the best form of treatment. The ultimate effect of this strategy was a dramatic decrease in overall drug consumption in general and cocaine use in particular. The specifics of these demand reduction efforts will be discussed in later chapters.

- An estimated 23 million people were current illegal drug users in 1985; 6 years later, in 1991, this number had decreased to 12.6 million.
- Current cocaine users—people who had used the drug within the previous month—fell from 5.8 million in 1985 to 1.9 million in 1991.
- Among high school seniors, 17.3% had tried cocaine in 1985; by 1991 this number had been cut to 7.8%.
- In 1985, approximately 30% of high school seniors admitted to using at least one illegal drug in the last month; by 1991 this number had dropped to 16.4%.
- In 1991, 93.9% of high school seniors disapproved of adults using cocaine even once or twice; in 1985 only 79.3% disapproved.

These findings establish that education leading to

prevention is the greatest deterrent to drug use. Figure 1.1 demonstrates how education can prevent drug use. This graph shows that drug declines when *perception* of cocaine's danger increases, an effect that occurs regardless of the reported availability of a drug.

The educational approach depends on a number of fundamental concepts, including the understanding that drug use is not caused by poverty or unemployment (the majority of poor and/or unemployed people do not use drugs), nor is it a product of race (most minority people do not use drugs). Rather, drug use results primarily from poor personal judgment: *The*

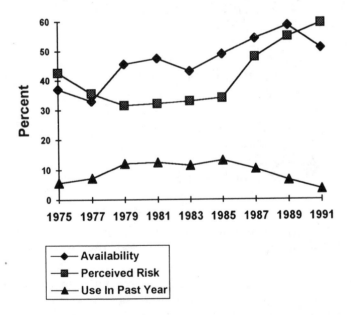

FIGURE 1.1. Trends in cocaine availability, perceived risk, and use in the past year for high school seniors. SOURCE: NIDA National High School Senior Survey, 1991.

user believes that the short-term pleasure outweighs the long-term cost of drug use. Clearly, a number of social factors, such as viable employment and stable familial structures, influence a person's decision not to use drugs. But education that accurately describes the long-term costs of drug use (addiction, health complications, loss of job and family, and so on) can effectively help individuals resist the short-term pleasures associated with drugs.

However, the educational approach does have limitations. Most notably, this strategy works best with the so-called recreational or casual user and with individuals who have employment and family supports. Individuals who are already experiencing significant drug use or who have limited employment and family resources do not respond as well. This population presents challenges different from that of the recreational user.

The findings of the 1991 National Household Survey supports this stratification of users. The dramatic decline in drug use reported in the late 1980s has slowed considerably.

As Figure 1.2 shows, a slight increase in monthly cocaine use occurred between 1990 and 1991 (from 0.8 to 0.9%). This increase results primarily from a surge in cocaine use by individuals age 35 and over. (Remove this age group and there is actually a 4% decrease in monthly cocaine use.) Two factors may explain the increase in drug use among the 35+ age group: the drug-using population and the high recividism among users. This increase is not surprising considering that some of the drug users who previously fell into younger groups have now migrated to the older group. It is

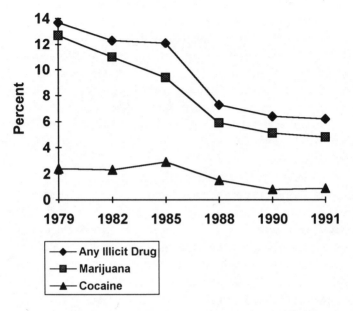

FIGURE 1.2. Past month's use of drugs. SOURCE: NIDA National Household Survey, 1991.

also possible that much of our recent antidrug efforts, concentrating on the vulnerable adolescent and young adult groups, need to be refocused on this older group.

The Persistence of Substance Abuse

The slight increase in cocaine use for the 35+ age group illustrates the entrenched nature of illegal drug use in America. Despite the recent success in curtailing drug use, there is little chance that the threats posed by drugs will subside. The powerful rewarding effects of drugs, the tendency for drug users to relapse, and a sophisticated illicit drug marketing and distribution network augurs against the imminent demise of illegal drug consumption. The complexity behind the reward and withdrawal effects of drugs makes the possibility of a "magic bullet" pharmacological treatment for addiction extremely remote. Similarly, the democratization of Europe and Russia opens up potentially lucrative markets for the drug trade and may be the latest development in cocaine distribution.

The Evolution of Cocaine Trafficking

In the late 1970s and early 1980s, cocaine use increased. Misleading reports surfaced about cocaine's supposedly nonaddictive nature and its ability to enhance sexual prowess and even work performance. This false information combined with cocaine's high expense and limited distribution to enhance cocaine's reputation as the "champagne" of illegal drugs. Cocaine became symbolic of the wealthy, jet-setting class. Although cocaine use did increase, its use was still mitigated somewhat by its cost. The advent of *crack* changed the economics and demographics of cocaine.

The first reported use of crack occurred in the Bahamas in 1983, but the widespread use of crack really began in 1985. Crack proved to be a drug marketeer's dream: a low initial cost combined with a highly addictive substance. Crack is actually the crystalline form of cocaine that occurs when powdered cocaine hydrochloride has been heated and then cooled. The name crack refers to the sound made when the crystallized cocaine is smoked.

The common perception of crack as a "pure"

and inexpensive form of cocaine is false. Crack is not unadulterated cocaine; any impurities in the powdered cocaine or substances used to "cut" or dilute the cocaine (such as baking soda or quinine) will appear in concentrated form in the crack crystals. Although the initial cost of crack certainly is less than that of a gram of powdered cocaine, the cumulative cost of crack surpasses that of powdered cocaine. For example, a $10 vial of crack contains approximately 100 mg of cocaine, which translates into $100 per gram. Conversely, cocaine powder normally sells for well under $100 per gram.

In the 1980s, cocaine distribution was largely controlled by the Medellín cartel, named for a city in Colombia. The brazenly violent tactics of this cartel, murdering hundreds of Colombian judges and government officials and terrorizing the streets and citizens of the major U.S. cities, allowed the Medellín faction to gain control of the cocaine trade. But the notoriety of these violent attacks also helped to mobilize the governments of both the United States and Colombia to launch a counterattack. These efforts have led to the systematic dismantling of the Medellín cartel, culminating in the June 1991 arrest of Pablo Escobar Gaviria, the chief of the Medellín faction.

Unfortunately, an even more powerful and sinister faction, the Cali cartel, has surfaced. In 1991, the Drug Enforcement Administration (DEA) estimated that the Cali cartel produced 70% of the cocaine entering the United States. The Cali faction is so strong that Robert Bonner, administrator of the DEA, labels them as "the most powerful criminal organization in the world. No drug organization rivals them today or perhaps anytime in history."[5] Unlike the Medellín cartel, the Cali organization eschews violence whenever possible, pre-ferring a more professional and low-key profile.

Recently, the Cali cartel has focused on the grow-ing drug markets in Europe and Japan. This faction already controls approximately 90% of the drugs enter-ing Europe. Cali-associated bank accounts have been uncovered in Hungary, Israel, and throughout Western Europe. The DEA reports that the Cali cartel is eagerly attempting to infiltrate Japan, where the current price of cocaine can reach $65,000 per kilogram.[5]

Law enforcement, fighting back against the Cali faction, has succeeded in dismantling a number of Cali distribution rings and in arresting a number of their prominent leaders. However, the Cali cartel appears to be more organized and entrenched than the Medellín and will most likely require a significant expenditure in time and money to be defeated.

The difficult task of confronting the illegal drug trade has led some individuals to propose legalization of drugs. Although legalization may appear to be a "quick fix," the increased drug use that would accom-pany legalization would present problems (addiction and addiction-related illnesses, accidents, and so on) far worse than our current situation. Furthermore, there is the distinct possibility that the illicit drug trade would continue to be profitable even with legalization. (The legalization of drugs will be discussed in greater detail in the next chapter.)

Remaining Challenges

Clearly the problems posed by cocaine are not likely to disappear soon. As a result, the physician's role in the antidrug effort should not be overlooked. This book is an attempt to help physicians and psychiatrists to stress both the detection and the prevention of drug abuse in their practice. Subsequent chapters provide the clinician with the latest information covering the medical and psychiatric complications of cocaine use, as well as the most current data regarding the neurobiological and psychosocial aspects of reward, withdrawal, and addiction. The pharmacological and nonpharmacological management of addiction, in inpatient, outpatient, and follow-up settings, is also discussed. Additional emphasis is placed on the detection and prevention of drug abuse via drug testing and educational efforts. It is fervently hoped that the information in this book will provide physicians with a valuable tool in the understanding, treatment, and prevention of cocaine abuse.

References

1. National Institute on Drug Abuse. *The National Household Survey on Drug Abuse.* Rockville, Md; December 1991.
2. National Institute on Drug Abuse. *The National High School Senior Survey.* Rockville, Md; February 1992.
3. Phibbs CS, Bateman DA, Schwartz RM. The neonatal costs of maternal cocaine use. *J Am Med Assoc.* 1991; 266(11):1521–1526.
4. National Institute on Drug Abuse. *Recent Hospital Emergency Room Data from the Drug Abuse Warning Network (DAWN).* Rockville, Md; December 1991.
5. Shannon, E. New kings of coke. *Time.* July 1, 1991:29–36.

2

The History of Cocaine

Cocaine derives from the leaves of coca plants—*Erythroxylon coca*—which are indigenous to South America. Use of coca leaves may date as far back as 5000 years before the Christian era. Burial sites from 2500 BCE in what is now Peru reveal coca leaves apparently stockpiled to assist the dead in their afterlife.[1] Archaeologists have also found evidence that by 1500 BCE our ancestors may have used a liquid coca-leaf compound as an anesthetic during brain surgery. The Incan word for the coca plant, *kuka*, is the antecedent of our word *coca*.

Coca played a major role in the religion of the Incan empire (13th–16th centuries). Coca was considered a sacred plant that was originally a gift from the first Inca. Coca leaves were used as talismans, or good luck charms, and played an integral part in many religious ceremonies. At that time, the coca leaf was chewed with lime to help bind the coca leaf, to as-

11

sist the high priest's meditative states, and to enhance the coca leaf's stimulant abilities. Pre-Colombian artifacts, some over 3000 years old, show men with bulging cheeks that are most likely filled with cocaine.[1]

Prior to the Spanish Conquest, laborers of the northern Andes chewed coca leaves while mining tin and silver and while working in the fields. These workers used coca chewing to offset the hypoxia that occurs in high altitudes and to overcome the fatigue of working long hours. Chewing coca leaves was so common that when the explorer Amerigo Vespucci came to the New World in the 15th century, he found Indians with bulging cheeks that reminded him of cattle.[2]

Following the Conquest, the Church initially tried to ban coca leaf, primarily because of its religious associations. This ban failed and the Spanish leaders eventually encouraged coca leaf chewing as a means of increasing the productivity of their Indian laborers. Coca chewing did little for the health of the workers: According to skeletal remains, the life span of the Indian laborer barely exceeded 30 years.

The coca leaf chewing of the Indians is actually an inefficient means of absorbing cocaine. Researchers have suggested that the average user chewed 60 grams of coca leaves a day.[3] Given that the alkaloid content of a cocaine leaf is about 0.5 to 0.7% and that only a portion of the alkaloid is absorbed in digestion, the total dosage would have been 200 to 300 mg spread over a 24-hour period. The effects associated with one episode of chewing coca leaves have been compared to consuming two cups of coffee.

The ancient practice of cocaine chewing has persisted through the years and is still reputed to allay hunger, overcome mountain sickness, negate cold temperatures (via blood vessel constriction and the heat generated by increased heart and muscle contraction), and even stifle stomach pains. The coca chewer does not feel euphoric, and reportedly the mountain laborers either reduce or eliminate their coca chewing after resettlement in the valleys.[1] The experience of the coca leaf chewing Indians highlights the importance of the route of administration on the rate of addiction and the severity of side effects. Today, the same Indians whose ancestors chewed coca leaves now suffer from crack addiction.

The Cocaine "Miracle" of the 19th Century

In 1859, a German scientist named Albert Niemann extracted the primary alkaloid from coca leaves and named this alkaloid cocaine. Soon reports wildly trumpeted cocaine's miraculous powers and ability to overcome fatigue. An Italian neurologist, Dr. Paola Montegazza, even wrote that "God is unjust because he made man incapable of sustaining the effect of coca all life long."[1]

In the early 1880s, these reports came to the attention of a young Sigmund Freud. Freud was searching for a research project that would bring him fame and enough money to marry. Cocaine seemed like the perfect solution, since at that time a condition called neurasthenia, or nervous exhaustion, was very common in Vienna. Freud began by administering cocaine to himself, to his fiancée, and to his patients. The preliminary results proved both very promising and misleading.

In 1884, Freud published his famous paper *Über*

Coca, in which he praised cocaine as a treatment for depression, nervousness, morphine addiction, alcoholism, digestive disorders, and even asthma. Freud wrote that "even repeated doses of cocaine produced no compulsive desire to use the stimulant further; on the contrary one feels a certain unmotivated aversion to the substance."[4]

Freud administered cocaine to his friend Dr. Ernst von Fleishl-Marxow, to treat the pain resulting from his friend's amputation and his subsequent addiction to morphine.[5] Soon Fleishl began using increasing amounts of subcutaneously injected cocaine. He became paranoid, suffered from delusions, and quickly became unmanageable.

Contemporaries of Freud also began experimenting with cocaine in the 1880s. In 1887, William Hammond, a prominent neurologist and former Surgeon General of the United States, spoke glowingly of cocaine and stated emphatically that cocaine was no more addictive than coffee or tea. Soon Dr. Hammond began a series of subcutaneous cocaine injections, starting with 65 mg and increasing the dose each day. Increased side effects, ranging from headaches to loss of mental control to severe cardiac and respiratory side effects, accompanied the increased doses. After only 6 days, Hammond reached a dosage level that would have been fatal if intravenously injected.[1]

Angelo Mariani, a chemist from Corsica, bottled and sold a cocaine-containing drink called Vin Mariani. The label on a bottle of Vin Mariani proclaimed that it prevented malaria, influenza, and "wasting diseases." Thomas Edison and Pope Leo XIII were enthusiastic supporters of the product.[6]

The *New York Times* echoed the cocaine excitement of that era. The September 2, 1885 edition of the *Times* stated, "The new uses to which cocaine has been applied with success in New York include hay fever, catarrh and toothache, and it is now being experimented with in cases of seasickness . . . . Cocaine will cure the worst cold in the head ever heard of."[1]

The Parke-Davis pharmaceutical company declared that cocaine was potentially "the most important therapeutic discovery of the age" and began selling cocaine-containing products, such as coca cigarettes used to treat throat infections. Cocaine was promoted as a cure for everything from seasickness and tired blood to hemorrhoids.

In 1886, John Pemberton, a pharmacist from Atlanta, created a drink, "Coca-Cola," made from a secret formula of coca leaves, kola nuts, and a small amount of cocaine in a sugary carbonated syrup. Originally this syrup was a prescription product recommended for hysteria, headache, and melancholia. In 1891, Asa Chandler obtained the secret formula and founded the Coca-Cola Company. Until 1904, the syrup was sold at soda fountains and promoted as a restorative tonic. (After that time the company, reacting to public pressure, removed cocaine from its formula.)[7]

The First Cocaine "Crash"

The euphoria surrounding cocaine in the 1880s soon dissipated. Soon, evidence mounted against the original claims of cocaine's safety. Hundreds of reports surfaced detailing addiction, psychotic behavior, convulsions, and deaths that were caused by cocaine. People realized that the feelings of power and euphoria that initially accompany cocaine deteriorated with repeated use into feelings of powerlessness and profound depression.

Even a patient of Freud's overdosed on cocaine. Freud later referred to 1885 as the "least successful and darkest year of my life." By 1887, only 3 years after his initial infatuation, Freud admitted in a paper entitled "Craving For and Fear of Cocaine" that cocaine produced paranoia, hallucination, and physical and mental deterioration.

The public, responding to these reports, pressured their elected officials to take action. In a recent article, David Musto aptly described the American mood in the late 1800s when he wrote:

> In a spirit not unlike that of our times, Americans in the last decade of the 19th century grew increasingly concerned about the environment, adulterated foods, destruction of the forests and the widespread use of mood-altering drugs.[8]

As a result, the federal government, despite the opposing efforts of pharmaceutical companies, instituted the Pure Food and Drug Act of 1906. Before this act, manufacturers did not have to list the ingredients in their products. Because there was no regulation, a wide variety of ingredients, including alcohol, cocaine, and morphine, could be used in these patent medicines regardless of whether they had any therapeutic benefit. The 1906 Pure Food and Drug Act attempted to change this by calling for accurate labeling of all patent remedies sold interstate, but it did *not* prevent sales of either cocaine or opiates. The problems of cocaine addiction and the violence associated with it continued to plague America.[8]

In 1907, New York State, in an attempt to curtail its open-market abuse, placed cocaine's availability directly under a physician's control. Even though cocaine could be legally obtained from a physician, the "black market" sale of cocaine thrived in New York. Musto reported that in 1907 the street price of cocaine was 25 cents a packet (from 65 to 130 mg of cocaine). Even though this price, about the equivalent of the average laborer's hourly wage, was significantly less than the cost of physician-obtained cocaine, it still maintained a healthy profit margin for the street dealers.

In 1910, President William Howard Taft submitted a report to Congress that stated that cocaine was the worst drug problem that had ever confronted America. Public pressure to limit cocaine and other mood-altering substances increased.

These pressures posed difficult questions for our legislators. How could federal law interfere with a physician's practice or a pharmacist's record keeping? The legislators hit on a brilliant solution: taxes. The Harrison Act of 1914 required a strict monitoring of the process behind coca or opiate products entering this country and ultimately reaching the patient. At each step in the process a tax was applied and Treasury Department permits were required. Individual patients were simply not granted permits. Furthermore, the Harrison Act limited cocaine to a prescription-only basis and forbade its inclusion in any nonprescription product (opiates were still allowed in nonprescription products such as cough medicine). The restrictions against cocaine were the strongest ever applied to any addictive drug.

The Decline of Cocaine Use

Public anger at the problems caused by cocaine combined with enforcement of the Harrison Act to significantly reduce cocaine consumption after 1914. By 1930 the New York City Mayor's Committee went so far as to proclaim that "during the last 20 years cocaine as an addiction has ceased to be a problem." By the 1930s, the therapeutic uses of cocaine had dwindled to the point where cocaine was used only as a topical anesthetic. The illegal use of cocaine was basically limited to the small percentage of the wealthy upper class who could afford the drug.

While cocaine use declined dramatically, users turned to amphetamines and other central nervous system stimulants that were first developed in the 1930s. Users report that the effects of cocaine and amphetamines are virtually indistinguishable, with the possible exception that the high from amphetamines lasts longer. On the surface, the longer high from amphetamines would appear to make this drug more appealing to users. Yet, on the street, users consider cocaine to be superior. Apparently, the shorter high makes cocaine more reinforcing and therefore more addictive. Amphetamines not only produce a similar euphoria, but the physical changes—such as increased heart rate, elevated blood pressure, and sweating—are almost identical.

Unfortunately, amphetamines also share cocaine's penchant for fatalities. By the late 1960s, drug users recognized the danger in amphetamines, hence the contemporary slogan "Speed Kills." Eventually, amphetamines were listed as a controlled substance, making them more difficult to obtain.

The 1960s

To fully understand the cocaine epidemic of the late 1970s, one must comprehend how the 1960s created an atmosphere conducive to drug experimentation. Before the 1960s, the single greatest factor that limited drug abuse was the public abhorrence of drugs. Popular movies portrayed drug users as obvious junkies who were symbolic of moral and physical failure. During the turmoil of the 1960s, people questioned not only the specifics of the Vietnam War, racism, and pollution but even the values of a society that would allow these problems to exist. The values of the older generation were routinely scorned and ridiculed as the youth of America considered the majority of people over the age of 30 to be morally and spiritually dead. The younger generation exerted a tremendous pressure to change society that did not end with antiwar rallies or civil rights marches but instead encompassed every element of society from hair length, clothes, and music to promiscuous sex, rampant drug use, and widespread revolution.

Drugs became so intertwined with the social and political issues of the 1960s that using drugs became "normal" and acceptable behavior. Some people viewed drug use as a conduit to a higher consciousness and greater spirituality. Those who refused to use drugs were regarded as part of the establishment responsible for Vietnam, racism, and pollution.

Without question, the primary illegal drug of that era was marijuana. In general, marijuana acts as a central nervous system depressant. Whenever a drug of a particular class, for example a depressant like marijuana, becomes popular, there is frequently a subsequent increase in drugs that have the *opposite* effect (that is, stimulants).

Drug users searching for a stimulant soon rediscovered cocaine. In the early to late 1970s, cocaine abuse increased, especially among middle- and upper-middle-class populations. In 1977, *Newsweek* reported that cocaine was becoming a mainstay of the most fashionable parties.[6] In a popular movie of that time, Woody Allen had his character make what was considered a major faux pas: sneezing into a pile of cocaine that was being freely distributed at a party. During the late 1970s, cocaine was the big "in joke" on TV's "Saturday Night Live." The warnings of cocaine's dangers from the 19th-century epidemic had long since been forgotten.

During the 1970s, cocaine was usually administered intranasally. A typical user bought a gram of cocaine for approximately $150 and snorted the drug from a tiny "coke spoon" or through a straw. The coke spoon method delivered between 5 and 10 mg of the drug. A "line" of cocaine inhaled through a straw delivered approximately 25 mg. Typical users would repeat the dose in both nostrils, thus taking between 10 and 50 mg of cocaine at a time.

The medical literature of the late 1970s and early 1980s ignored the lessons that had been learned almost 100 years earlier and instead contributed to the typical user's perception that cocaine was safe and nonaddicting. For example, an article published in 1977 claimed that aside from the cost, "the main undesirable effects of 'social snorting' are nervousness, irritability, and restlessness from overstimulation."[9] The authors,

Grinspoon and Bakalar, went on to state that cocaine may improve physical performance, cure stage fright, and fortify the body and mind without the risk of causing a withdrawal syndrome marked by prolonged cravings for the drugs. The same authors, writing in the 1980 edition of the *Comprehensive Textbook of Psychiatry*, stated: "Used no more than two or three times a week, cocaine creates no serious problems. In daily and fairly large amounts, it can produce minor psychological disturbances. Chronic cocaine abuse usually does not appear as a medical problem."[10]

Obviously, these statements did little to discourage drug use. As the demand for cocaine grew, the supply of cocaine rose, the price dropped, and the amount of a typical dose increased. The increasing availability changed the demographic patterns of cocaine use. A survey of cocaine users conducted in 1983 found that half of the users had at least some college education and that 52% were earning more than $25,000 a year.[6]

Such findings confirmed the image of cocaine as the drug of choice among the elite. As a "status" drug, cocaine seduced intelligent, competent people perhaps because it temporarily enhanced the qualities we associate with achievement. Cocaine users reported having more energy, less need for sleep, enhanced self-esteem, and high ambition—all the skills deemed essential by high-powered executives.

Before 1985, less than half of the callers in a national survey reported using cocaine daily—most took it only a few times a week. It is important to note that even at this relatively low intake, 63% of those surveyed considered themselves addicted. Over 70% stated that they preferred cocaine to food, and half would rather use the drug than have sex. One out of 10 reported that they had attempted suicide. The addiction process associated with cocaine appears to be accelerated.[6]

The Evolution of Cocaine Use

A new method of cocaine administration called "freebasing" allowed users to smoke the drug and absorb much higher doses than ever before. Freebase is smokable cocaine obtained by dissolving the white crystalline powder, cocaine hydrochloride, in a strong base. Smoking coke gives a quicker, more intense high than inhaling cocaine powder because the drug passes quickly and unhindered from the lungs to the bloodstream. The process of freebasing cocaine can be dangerous: For example, the comedian Richard Pryor was badly burned when the ether he used to process cocaine exploded.

The arrival of the crack form of cocaine in the mid-1980s signaled a major escalation in the problems associated with cocaine abuse. Freebase cocaine was essentially mass-produced, and the low initial cost of crack made it available to younger users and sent the average age of the user spiraling downward. Causing users to feel more powerful, more confident, more intelligent, and more in control, smoked cocaine is rapidly addicting and produces medical effects previously seen only in long-term intranasal users. By 1987, 56% of callers to a national hotline reported that they were smoking their cocaine; just 4 years earlier, only 21% said they were freebasing.

Within two decades, what was considered a

"dose" of cocaine changed significantly. Higher doses of more potent cocaine have transformed the experience of the drug and its impact on society tremendously. For example, a study of drug use by male arrestees in large metropolitan areas found that over 50% tested positive for cocaine (see Figure 2.1).

In addition, drug dealers have sought new products or product combinations that would entice their consumers. One new product, a stimulant with cocainelike effects called "Ice," has recently received much attention (see Chapter 10 for more information).

Other Forms of Cocaine

New methods of administering cocaine are continually evolving. By packaging crude cocaine with marijuana or tobacco, drug dealers have created a highly addictive drug called *bazuco* or *bazooka*. Some users mix

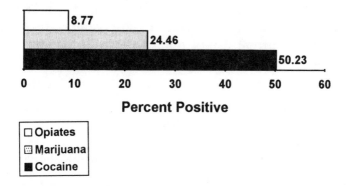

FIGURE 2.1. Rates of drug use by male arrestees in 13 large metropolitan areas. SOURCE: National Institute of Justice/Drug Use Forecasting Program, January through March 1989.

cocaine with heroin to offset the unpleasant stimulant effects, to extend the euphoria, and to help control the postcocaine withdrawal. This combination, known as the speedball, killed John Belushi. Close to 90% of cocaine users also use some other form of drug, especially depressants such as alcohol, marijuana, and heroin.

The Rise of Polydrug Abuse

Several studies have confirmed the comorbidity of various substances of abuse. The Epidemiological Catchment Area (ECA) study found that 16% of the general population experienced alcoholism at some point during their lifetime. Thirty percent of these alcoholics also suffered from other drug dependence. Similarly, the rates of alcohol dependence among other drug addicts were high: 36% of cannabis addicts, 62% of amphetamine addicts, 67% of opiate addicts, and 84% of cocaine addicts were also alcoholics.[11] These studies, combined with clinical observations regarding the concurrent use of multiple substances, suggest common biological determinants while complicating treatment.[12]

The Success of Antidrug Campaigns

No history of cocaine in America would be complete without a chronicling of the recent success in curtailing drug use. The antidrug effort that began in the mid-1980s has demonstrated that sound information, clearly communicated, is an extremely effective weapon in the war against drugs. The drop in the current users of cocaine from 5.8 million in 1985 to 1.4 million in 1991 illustrates how *effective education prevents drug abuse.* Many schools, businesses, and families realistically emphasized the dangers of drugs.

Schools across the country added drug education programs, while employee assistance programs aimed at helping the drug-abusing employee grew rapidly in the 1980s. Employee drug testing, once so obscure that a 1982 government publication on employee drug abuse failed to mention the subject, became a major factor in employer efforts to prevent drug-using applicants from joining the company and to improve the safety and productivity of the company. In addition, public service announcements—many created by the highly effective Partnership for a Drug-Free America—reached many segments of our population.

The new antidrug campaign wisely focused on the reduction of *all* drug use. By avoiding messages directed specifically at individual drugs, the campaign eluded the confusion and expense that frequently appear following repeated efforts to establish new drug targets and goals. The broad-based campaign has the added benefit of addressing the people who abuse multiple drugs. This problem of multiple drug abuse is so common that one major study of the general population, the Epidemiologic Catchment Area Study, recently found that 84% of cocaine addicts also suffered from alcoholism.

The success of the antismoking campaign has served as an excellent model for the antidrug campaign. In the early 1960s, who could have predicted that the antismoking movement would create smoke-free offices, airplanes, restaurants, and hotel rooms? Public education about the dangers of smoking and passive inhalation of smoke changed attitudes about smoking. Before the 1960s it was considered impolite not to offer your friend a cigarette if you wanted to smoke; today, it is considered impolite to smoke without first requesting permission.

The antidrug campaign has witnessed a similar change in attitudes. In the 1970s it was almost impossible to attend a concert or sporting event without witnessing blatant substance abuse. Today, many stadiums have family sections where all drug use (even alcohol consumption) is strictly banned.

Changes in Youth Attitudes

Since 1987, the Partnership for a Drug-Free America has played an integral role in helping to change American attitudes. The Partnership, an organization using many of this country's best advertising and marketing minds, has created a remarkable series of advertisements aimed at "unselling" drugs. These ads, in a direct and powerful manner, demystify and deglamorize drug use. While these ads have helped to reduce drug use in general, they have had an especially significant effect on youth.

Surveys of adolescents conducted for the Partnership[13] have shown that educational efforts can foster antidrug attitudes in a very short period of time. For example:

- From 1987 to 1991, the percentage of adolescents (age 13–17) who agreed with the statement "I don't want to hang around people who use drugs" increased from 54 to 64%.

- The percentage of adolescents who agreed with the statement "People who try drugs act stupidly and foolishly" increased from 64% in 1987 to 69% in 1991.
- In 1987, 73% of adolescents believed that "drugs make you do worse at school, work, or athletics, etc." In 1991, this number had increased to 78%.
- Sixty-six percent of adolescents agreed in 1987 with the statement "Taking drugs scares me." In 1991, this percentage had increased to 74%.

These changes in attitudes have affected usage rates. In 1985, 17.3% of high school seniors had tried cocaine; by 1991, this number had declined 55% to 7.8%.[14] Clearly, as the antidrug atmosphere increases, drug use decreases.

Changes in Adult Attitudes

Adults have also been affected by the antidrug campaign:

- The number of adults who disagreed with the statement "People who try drugs are adventurous" increased from 61% in 1987 to 71% in 1990.
- Sixty-seven percent of adults disagreed in 1987 with the statement "Using cocaine is a status symbol." By 1990, this number had increased to 73%.
- The percentage of adults who thought that a

cocaine user "has no future" increased from 56% in 1987 to 63% in 1990.
- From 1987 to 1990, the percentage of adults who believed that a cocaine user was "a loser" increased from 50 to 56%.

Corresponding with this increasingly negative view of drug users was a sharp decline in the number of current cocaine users, from an estimated 5.8 million in 1985 to 1.4 million in 1991.

Remaining Challenges

The positive signs of declining drug use are tempered by signs that indicate that the threat of drug abuse still remains significant. Aside from the increase in cocaine use by the 35+ age group detailed in Chapter 1, a recent Partnership survey found that:

- Ten percent of children 9 to 12 years old said that it was easy to get cocaine or crack.
- Fifteen percent of these preteens report that they have been asked to buy or use drugs.
- Twenty percent of children 9 to 12 years old admitted to using alcohol and/or cigarettes.

Other surveys have found that:

- In 1990, 5 million junior and senior high school students were classified as "binge drinkers," with 500,000 students bingeing at least once a week.
- In 1991, an estimated 18% of all high school seniors were daily cigarette smokers. (Cigarette

smoking is a major risk factor for future illegal drug use.)

- Ten percent of all babies born in the United States were exposed to at least one illegal drug while in the womb.

In addition to these statistics, recent efforts to legalize drugs may help to create an atmosphere, perhaps inadvertently, that diminishes the dangers associated with drug use. Legalization implies safety (no matter how many warnings appear on the label). Figure 1.1 (in Chapter 1) depicts the increased drug use that occurs when the perceived risk of drugs decreases, and there is reason to believe that legalization will diminish the perception of cocaine's danger.

The Legalization Debate

Recently, a significant number of politicians, lawyers, and political commentators have supported the legalization of cocaine and heroin. Basically, the pro-legalization proposition can be divided into four points.

The first point can be summarized as, "Nothing can stop drug use; therefore, why not try legalization?" This logic fails because it ignores our recent success in dramatically reducing the number of drug users. In 1990, nearly 90% of high school seniors disapproved of cocaine use, and in just 1 year the proportion of them who used cocaine dropped 20%. Among the population as a whole, use of all illicit drugs decreased 37%.

The second point states, "Legalization won't increase the number of addicts." Surveys sponsored by the Partnership find repeatedly that the greatest deterrent to drug use is fear—fear of getting caught, fear of punishment, fear of harm. Without legal sanctions against drugs, we lose a key defensive weapon.

The third point—"Tobacco and alcohol are legal, why not other drugs?"—focuses on an apparent contradiction. Tobacco and alcohol cause nearly 500,000 deaths a year, plus other illnesses, accidents, and birth defects. Right now illicit drugs cause approximately 6000 deaths a year.

Those favoring legalized drugs argue that Prohibition failed to stop drinking. In reality, Prohibition reduced drinking by one-third and produced a 64% drop in deaths from cirrhosis and a 53% decline in admissions to mental hospitals. Alcohol and cigarettes have been a deadly part of American life for at least 300 years; adding more potentially dangerous drugs would only increase morbidity and mortality. Most Americans insist prescription medications undergo years of safety testing before we let people take them; we should certainly insist on the same process for illicit drugs before declaring them safe.

The final point states, "Legalization means less crime." According to this theory, less crime will result for two reasons. First if addicts can easily purchase cocaine, they won't have to commit crimes to purchase their drugs. Second, legalization will put drug dealers out of business and eliminate the violent crimes associated with their trade. The first point ignores the true nature of cocaine-related crime: The majority of cocaine-related crimes are committed while the user is using cocaine. In the first quarter of 1989, 76% of all people arrested in New York City had cocaine in their urine, even though cocaine is quickly eliminated from the body.

The second point assumes that legalization would eliminate the criminal activity associated with drugs. It is likely that there will always be a black market for illegal drugs like cocaine. What law-abiding and tax-paying corporation could compete with underground cartels whose profits are not reduced by having to pay health care benefits for their employees?

Finally, if legalization did occur, we would still have to find a way to limit the purchases of cocaine, since users report virtually no tolerance to the drug and since cocaine demands consumption of ever-increasing amounts. Many difficult questions remain unresolved: for example, How much cocaine can a user buy a day? If we allow users to buy 1 gram they will soon demand 2 or more grams—and even that amount will not be enough.

Proponents of legalization frequently ignore that America has already experimented with legalized drugs. One hundred years ago, all drugs, including cocaine and heroin, were legal. The American people found this legalized state so abhorrent that they demanded that our government embark on the then revolutionary path of making these drugs illegal. Even the 1907 New York State attempt to make cocaine powder available only on a prescription basis failed because the black market could offer far cheaper cocaine—a result that would most likely happen today if crack and heroin were made prescription drugs.

A Discussion with Robert DuPont, M.D.

The following discussion with Robert DuPont, M.D., one of this country's leading drug abuse experts, provides an interesting and personal perspective on the legalization debate.

Q: *Should drugs be legalized?*
A: Unfortunately, I have a personal—and somewhat embarrassing—story regarding decriminalization, a close relative of legalization. In the 1970s, I was appointed White House "Drug Czar" under Richard Nixon. At that time, President Nixon told me that I could comment publicly on any aspect of our nation's drug policy except one: Under no circumstances could I support the legalization or decriminalization of marijuana. This seemed like a reasonable request and I agreed to this condition. Legalization means that the sale and the use of a drug are legal. Decriminalization is a legal no-man's land where the sale of the drug remains a criminal offense.

A few years later, after Gerald Ford replaced Nixon in the White House, I continued to serve as Drug Czar. Since Nixon had left, I was no longer bound to remain silent on decriminalization. So, at a national press conference, I spoke in favor of decriminalization of marijuana. Although I never supported the legalization of marijuana or any other illegal drug, in 1975 I was convinced that decriminalization was the way of the future.

I watched, first with chagrin, and then with increasing horror, as marijuana use soared. In 1976, the number of high school seniors who were daily marijuana smokers was 6%. In 1978, this number rose to 11%. The percentage of *daily* marijuana smokers had nearly *doubled* in the three years after I spoke in favor of decriminalization.

By 1977, I had changed my position on decriminalization. Ironically, in 1977 President Carter—a supporter of decriminalization—replaced Ford in the White House. I was still Director of the National Institute on Drug Abuse, but now I was under orders *not* to speak out against decriminalization! As soon as I left the government in 1978, I admitted publicly that I made a mistake when I spoke in favor of decriminalization. Fortunately, 1978 was the high point for daily marijuana use (by 1990 it had declined to just over 2%).

By speaking out in favor of decriminalization while I was the government's top doctor dealing with drug abuse, I believe I contributed to the perception that drugs were not harmful. We now know that the perception of harmfulness may be the single most effective deterrent to drug use, even in the face of widely available drugs.

Q: *Many people say that cocaine and marijuana should be legalized because alcohol and tobacco are legal. What is your response to this?*
A: A major reason legalization should not be tried is that prohibition works! Consider alcohol, cigarettes, marijuana, and cocaine—the four most common drugs in America. In 1991, the total number of Americans, 12 years and older who have used the following drugs at least once in the previous 30 days are:

Alcohol:	103,232,000
Cigarettes:	54,805,000
Marijuana:	9,000,000
Cocaine:	1,892,000

Now let me give you the approximate numbers for the 1985 national survey:

Alcohol:	113,000,000
Cigarettes:	60,000,000
Marijuana:	18,000,000
Cocaine:	6,000,000

Between 1985 and 1991, the percentage of Americans using alcohol dropped around 8%. The percentage using cigarettes dropped 10%. But the percentage using marijuana dropped 50%, and the percentage using cocaine dropped 66%! Look at those numbers and tell me that prohibition is not working today. The two most common illegal drugs, marijuana and cocaine, are used by 9 and 2 million people, respectively. The
(continued)

legal drugs, alcohol and cigarettes, are used by 103 and 64 million, respectively. Think what would happen if cocaine and marijuana were treated like alcohol and cigarettes. Consider also that the social costs of alcohol (i.e., increased medical costs caused by alcoholism, lost productivity, more accidents, etc.) exceed the social cost of all illegal drugs put together. And if that isn't enough to convince you, consider that the deaths caused by cigarette smoking exceed the deaths by all illegal drugs plus alcohol put together.

Now think of those numbers and tell me that alcohol and tobacco look like good models for social policy for other addictive drugs. They look to me like models for absolute disaster.

Source: Adapted with permission from MS Gold (Ed.), The University of Florida's *Facts About Drugs and Alcohol Newsletter* 1(3), 1992.

References

1. Cohen S. *Cocaine Today.* Rockville, Md: American Council for Drug Education; 1981.
2. Brain PF, Coward GA. A review of the history, actions, and legitimate uses of cocaine. *J Substance Abuse.* 1989; 1:431–451.
3. Phillips J, Wynne RD. *Cocaine: The Mystique and the Reality.* New York: Avon Books; 1980.
4. Freud S. Über coca (On cocaine). In: Byck R, ed. *Cocaine Papers.* New York: Stonehill Publishing Co; 1974: 49–73.
5. Nasah GG. *Cocaine: The Great White Plague.* Middlebury, Vt: Paul S. Ericksson, Publishers; 1989.
6. Gold MS. *The Good News About Drugs and Alcohol.* New York: Villard Books; 1991.
7. Kahn EJ. *The Big Drink: The Story of Coca-Cola.* New York: Random House; 1960.
8. Musto D. Opium, cocaine, and marijuana in American history. *Scientific Am.* July 1991: 40–47.
9. Grinspoon L, Bakalar JB. A kick from cocaine. *Psychology Today* 1977; 10, 41–42, 78.

10. Grinspoon L, Bakalar JB. Drug dependence: Nonnarcotic agents. In: Kaplan HI, Freedman AM, Sadock BJ, eds. *Comprehensive Textbook of Psychiatry/III.* vol 2. Baltimore, Md: Williams & Wilkins; 1980: 1621.
11. Helzer, J, Burnam, A: Epidemiology of alcohol addiction: United States. In NS Miller (ed.), *Comprehensive Handbook of Drug and Alcohol Addiction.* Ch. 1, pp. 9–38. New York: Marcel Dekker; 1991.
12. Miller NS, Gold MS. Comorbidity of drug and alcohol addictions: Epidemiological, familial, and genetic evidence for common transmission. *American Journal on Addiction.* In press; 1992.
13. Black GS. The attitudinal basis of drug use 1987–1991. Reports from the Media-Advertising Partnership for a Drug-Free America, Inc. Gordon S. Black Corporation.
14. National Institute on Drug Abuse. *The National High School Senior Survey,* Rockville, Md., 1992.

3

The Neurobiology of Cocaine

The abuse and addiction potential of cocaine results, at least partly, from its effects on specific neurotransmitter systems of the brain. Recent laboratory research has established that cocaine and other drugs of abuse act directly on the brain's reward pathways. Although it may seem obvious that the euphoric effects of cocaine enhance the abuse potential of the drug, many attempts at understanding addiction have instead focused on etiologies other than endogenous reward, such as the self-medication theory. According to this theory, cocaine administration is an attempt to correct a major psychiatric problem such as depression. Although it is true that a psychological state like depression may be associated with the drug taking, cocaine itself is not an antidepressant. Furthermore, controlled studies have found that depressed or anxious people do not drink more than nondepressed or nonanxious individuals.[1]

Another theory, popular in the early 1980s, mistakenly centered on cocaine's relative lack of physical withdrawal symptoms as "proof" of cocaine's nonaddicting nature.[2] Cocaine was seen as a safe, nonaddicting means of experiencing euphoria. This perception combined with the dearth of clinical research on cocaine abuse to create an atmosphere conducive to cocaine experimentation. When reports of cocaine addiction soon surfaced in the mid-1980s, cocaine addiction was seen by many as a purely "psychological" and not physiological addiction. At that time, addiction and drug dependence were seen as resulting primarily from attempts to avoid the pain and discomfort associated with withdrawal.[3]

A more recent explanation focuses on cocaine's euphoric effect: Cocaine activates endogenous brain stimulation reward (BSR) neuroanatomical systems and thereby encourages repeated administration. While cocaine's effect on brain stimulation reward is complex, many studies have documented cocaine's ability to enhance dopamine release and levels at the synapse. Research indicates that these dopaminergic neural systems play an important part in rewarding effects associated with feeding, male sexual motivation, self-stimulation, drug use, and place-preference conditioning.[4] This endogenous positive reward system, accessed now by exogenous self-administration of cocaine, provides users with an experience that their brain equates with profoundly important events like eating, drinking, and sex.

Drug use soon becomes an acquired drive state that permeates all aspects of human life, potentially to the point where this new "drug drive" supersedes even basic survival drives. Withdrawal from drug use activates independent and separate neural pathways, which cause withdrawal events to be perceived as life threatening. The subsequent physiological and psychological reactions patients refer to as withdrawal symptoms also lead to drug consumption. This chapter discusses the neuroanatomical effects of cocaine compared to other drugs of abuse, with specific attention on how cocaine activates BSR, encourages repeated administration, and leads to its subtle withdrawal or abstinence state.

The Role of Reward in Drug Use

In the 1950s, researchers suggested that abuse-prone substances activated brain reward circuits.[5] Since that time, studies have confirmed that all substances of abuse:

- Either enhance brain stimulation reward or lower brain reward thresholds
- Affect brain reward circuits through either basal neuronal firing or basal neurotransmitter discharge
- Will cause animals to work for injections into the brain reward area but not for injections into other areas of the brain
- Will have their rewarding properties significantly mediated by blockades of the brain reward system through either lesions or pharmacological methods[6]

The medial forebrain bundle (MFB) region of the brain, together with the nuclei and projection fields of the MFB, has been found to be primarily responsible for the positive rewards associated with substance abuse. Histofluorescence mapping techniques revealed a close association between the brain stimulation reward region and the mesotelencephalic dopamine (DA) system.[7] Additional studies have confirmed the importance of DA neurotransmission to brain reward.[8,9] For example, selective DA receptor antagonists prevent cocaine self-administration by animals.[10] Although the initial hypothesis suggested that electrical brain stimulation reward directly triggered DA neurotransmission, it is now believed that the activation of the DA neurons occurs as a convergence following activation of a myelinated caudally running fiber system whose neurons lack the properties associated with DA neurons.[11] Drugs of abuse enhance brain stimulation reward primarily through their actions on this DA convergence.[12] Direct DA neurotransmission alone does not appear to be the sole basis for stimulant reward, since direct DA agonists such as apomorphine and piribedil, although self-administered by animals, are not self-administered to the same degree as indirect DA agonists that block the synaptic reuptake of DA.[13]

Electrical stimulation of the MFB can result in either positive or negative reinforcement. Positive reinforcement results from a stimulus that brings pleasure to a subject who is in a normal mood state. The identification of positive reinforcers is complicated by the highly subjective nature of pleasure and by the difficulties of defining normal mood states. Negative reinforcement is produced by the termination of dysphoria and the subsequent return to a normal state. Popular pain relievers such as aspirin and acetaminophen can be viewed as negative reinforcers.[14]

Species-specific survival drives, such as eating, drinking, copulating, and seeking shelter, are positive reinforcers. Drugs of abuse are also positive reinforcers. The fundamental element in animal response to these survival drives appears to be correlated with forward locomotion. In fact, the forward locomotion response apparently results from a number of drugs, including cocaine, amphetamines, opiates, barbiturates, benzodiazepines, alcohol, nicotine, caffeine, cannabis, and phencyclidine.[15] Specifically, these positive reinforcement drugs of abuse appear to share the common effect of enhancing DA levels (see Table 3.1).

Stimulant Reinforcement

Cocaine may achieve positive reinforcement by blocking the reuptake of DA into the presynaptic neuron.[15] By preventing DA reuptake, greater concentrations of DA remain in the synaptic cleft with more DA available at the postsynaptic site for stimulation of specific receptors. The abnormally high levels of DA in the synapse ultimately inhibit the firing rate of dopaminergic cells and forces more DA synthesis by blocking the process by which synaptic DA is inactivated and recycled[16] (see Table 3.2). Numerous studies have supported the positive reinforcement effects associated with increased synaptic levels of DA.[14] In animals, the electrical stimulation of the mesolimbic and/or mesocortical dopaminergic tracts produces reward-seeking behavior and increased extracellular DA levels similar to cocaine self-administration, while lesions in these tracts block

TABLE 3.1. Possible Neurochemical Basis for Reinforcement/
Withdrawal, with Associated Affective and Autonomic Withdrawal Levels

Abused Drugs	Reinforcement Effects	Withdrawal Effects	N Accumbens/ Affective Withdrawal	Locus Ceruleus/ Autonomic Withdrawal
Amphetamines	Enhanced DA Levels via presynaptic DA release	NE Depletion mutes LC hyperactivity	+++	++
Cocaine	Enhanced DA Levels via DA reuptake block	NE Depletion mutes LC hyperactivity	++++	++
Opiates	Increased DA firing	LC hyperactivity	++	++++
Marijuana	Enhanced DA levels via DA reuptake block	LC hyperactivity	++	++
Alcohol	Enhanced DA	LC hyperactivity	++	+++
Nicotine	Increased DA firing via nicotinic acetylcholine receptors	LC hyperactivity	+++	+

TABLE 3.2. Dopamine (DA) Disruptions Caused by Cocaine

Acute effects
  DA reuptake blockade (acute DA stimulation)
  Increased synaptic DA metabolism (acute DA depletion)
  Intraneuronal DA metabolism (acute DA depletion)

Chronic effects
  Decreased brain DA levels
  Increased DA binding sites (compensated depletion)
  Increased tyrosine hydroxylase activity (increased synthesis)
  Hyperprolactinemia (decreased DA functional tone)
  Decreased DA metabolism (homovanillic acid)

cocaine effects.[3] The DA surplus in turn activates responses along the sympathetic nervous system-producing such effects as vasoconstriction and acute increases in heart rate and blood pressure.[17,18]

The powerful rewarding aspects of cocaine have been illustrated by animal studies showing that cocaine is self-administered by animals to death[19] and is preferred over food, water, and sex.[20] Furthermore, a model for human reward can be found in the intracranial electrical self-stimulation (ICSS) of brain reward sites in animals. Chronic cocaine administration apparently increases ICSS reward threshold levels in DA reward areas and results in a down-regulation of the brain reward regions, an effect that correlates to the dysphoria associated with cocaine withdrawal. By interfering with neurochemical activity, cocaine acts in many ways like an artificially induced dopamine neurotransmitter. Table 3.3 lists many of the specific sites affected by cocaine.

Although the exact areas responsible for these reward regions are not certain, researchers have identi-

TABLE 3.3. Specific Sites Inhibited by Cocaine

Site	Yes	No	Maybe
Monoamine uptake	X		
D_1D_2	X		
$D_3D_4D_5$			X
5-HT	X		
Noradrenaline	X		
Neurotensin	X		
Opioid			X
Other peptides			X
CRF/ACTH			X
Other	X		

SOURCE: Woolverton WL, Johnson KM. Neurobiology of cocaine abuse. *TiPS* (13):193–200. May 1992.

fied seven different proteins that can act as dopamine receptors (D_{1a}, D_{1b}, D_{2short}, D_{2long}, D_3, D_4, D_5; see box below), all of which are distinct from the dopamine transporter(s). The assumption that cocaine binds to the dopamine transporter lies behind the dopamine hypothesis of cocaine reward. According to this theory, the dopamine transporter serves as the primary means of removing dopamine from the synaptic cleft after its release, and inhibition of this uptake results in an excess of dopamine in the synaptic cleft.[21] It has been hypothesized that the dopamine transporter is the cocaine receptor, that is, the initial site of action that ultimately leads to the reinforcement associated with the drug. The recent cloning of the dopamine transporter may someday lead to a greater understanding of the mechanisms mediating reward and addiction,[22] and the development of important and effective new treatments.

Cocaine's Behavioral Effects and Dopamine Receptors

In an attempt to better understand the role dopamine plays in cocaine's behavioral effects, recent research efforts have focused on the different types of dopamine receptors. Agonists of the D_2 receptor appear to have many cocainelike effects, such as locomotor activity, generation of stereotyped behavior, and positive reinforcement, while D_2 antagonists can inhibit some of the behavioral effects associated with cocaine.[88]

However, cocaine is more than a simple D_2 agonist since D_2 antagonists do not completely inhibit the stimulus effects of cocaine in animals or its subjective effects in humans. In addition, it is now apparent that the D_1 receptor plays a major role in the behavioral effects associated with cocaine. D_1 antagonists inhibit cocaine's effects, such as decreased food intake and increased locomotor activity.[88] As a result, D_1 antagonists may be effective in cocaine treatment. Further research is needed to better understand the role of all dopamine receptors in cocaine reward.

Serotonin and Other Factors in Stimulant Reward

One must caution against the overly simplistic view that cocaine's dopaminergic effects alone account for its reinforcing properties. Other factors, such as the serotonergic and opioid systems, most likely play an important role in BSR. For example, a recent study found that the opiate antagonist naltrexone attenuated cocaine self-administration in rats.[23] Cocaine's important opioid and serotonergic effects, in addition to DA augmentation, may explain why DA blockers like haloperidol are not as effective in cocaine reversal as naloxone is in blocking and reversing opioid effects.

Although the serotonin 5-HT uptake inhibitor flu-oxetine clearly reverses amphetamine self-administration, it is not effective in reversing cocaine self-administration. However, the serotonin $5-HT_2$ antagonist ritanserin has been found to reduce cocaine preference in rats. Apparently, ritanserin works on serotonergic systems and does not increase DA activity, nor interact with the behavioral responses triggered by cocaine. Furthermore, ritanserin's lack of abuse potential and its failure to affect food and/or fluid intake suggest that it affects the basic systems responsible for the need associated with cocaine reinforcement.[24] Additional findings confirming ritanserin's ability to reduce the intake and preference for alcohol and the opioid fentanyl, but not sucrose,[25] suggest some common involvement of $5-HT_2$ receptors in the reinforcement mechanism associated with drugs of abuse.

Nonpharmacological Factors

A recent rodent model for alcoholism provides an interesting example of some of the nonpharmacological factors in the development of addiction, including cocaine addiction.[26] In this model, different stages in the progression of addiction can be detected. First, rodents were given free and continuous choice of drinking either tap water or other solutions containing varying concentrations of ethanol (ETOH). During this phase the drug-taking behavior appeared to be exploratory: Days of high ETOH consumption were followed by days of abstinence. During this initial phase, the rodent developed a pattern of ETOH consumption that remained relatively constant for several months. Dose and consumption patterns were controlled at this time by a combination of environmental and individual factors. For example, socially isolated rats drank more ETOH than group-housed rodents. In addition, dominant rats drank nearly 50% less ETOH than their subordinates—a phenomenon that occurs even when the rats are socially isolated. (Wolffgramm has suggested that this phenomenon indicates that there may be a possible genetic disposition affecting both social dominance and drug preference.[26]) At this stage, levels of drug consumption can be reversed.

After approximately 6 months of continuous exposure to ETOH solutions, the rodents gradually adjusted their alcohol-taking behavior. Drug use gradually increased, although environmental factors remained constant. Previously, this increase had been attributed to the development of tolerance to the effects of ETOH. However, the author of this model observed no significant development of tolerance at this time—rather, the author attributed this increased consumption to increased demand for the drug.

Next, the author imposed a 9-month period (approximately one-third of the animals' life span) of abstinence from all ETOH solutions. Following this period of abstinence, the rodents were reintroduced to both tap water and ETOH fluids. They again displayed a strong preference for ETOH, a preference that persisted despite environmental changes (social isolation no longer affected consumption) and the addition of an aversive-tasting liquid to the ETOH solution. The authors defined this as a "behavioral dependence" on ETOH and considered it to be the equivalent of drug addiction in human beings.

The alcohol-dependent rodents displayed not only a lack of control over drug taking but also a change in the effects of ETOH. During the first phase of alcohol exposure, rodents were stimulated by low doses of ETOH and depressed by higher amounts. However, alcohol-dependent rats displayed the exact opposite effects: They were depressed by low doses and stimulated by high doses.

These alcohol-dependent rodents reflect the importance of the host in the development of addiction, and the study complements other research efforts that have succeeded in breeding rodent strains according to their preference for alcohol.[87] The alcohol-preferring (P) rats appear to be alcoholics: They voluntarily consume enough alcohol to cause inebriation even when there is sufficient food and water available. As with the Wolffgramm study, electroencephalograms (EEG) of P rats revealed that the P rats were stimulated by low doses of alcohol, whereas alcohol nonpreferring (NP) rats were mildly sedated by the alcohol.

In addition, the Wolffgramm study illustrates the importance of voluntary self-administration in the development of addiction. When ETOH was administered intragastrically, the differences between alcoholic and nonalcoholic rats were lessened. Route of administration, along with dose and type of drug, plays an essential role in the development of addiction. A central learning process, apparently occurring in the mesolimbic system, seemingly combines the rewarding effects of the drug with the voluntary self-administration and other environmental and social factors associated with the drug use to create a powerful "memory" or craving for the drug. Furthermore, this memory for the drug appears to be irreversible: 9 months of abstinence in rodents did not affect ETOH preference—a phenomenon that confirms the importance of life-long abstinence in human drug recovery.

The Physiological Aspects of Drug Memory

Recent research has centered on the role of the proto-oncogene c-*fos* in the central learning process underlying drug memory. These research efforts stem primarily from the attention devoted to understanding neural plasticity and the molecular process by which gene expression is altered, and from the specific molecular probes designed to study such phenomena. Concepts developed in oncogene research have been applied to the study of the nervous system, leading researchers to suggest that the transcription factors capable of oncogenic transformation and implicated in cell growth regulation also act as inducible transcription factors in the stimulus-response coupling in the nervous system.[27]

The majority of cell types have relatively low levels of c-*fos* and c-*jun*, the cellular homologues of the *fos* and *jun* oncogenes. Extracellular stimuli, however, will cause very high, transient levels of c-*fos* and c-*jun*.[28] The proto-oncogenes c-*fos* and c-*jun* are members of the set of genes called *cellular immediate-early genes*. Cellular immediate-early genes have been implicated in the coupling of short-term stimuli to long-term changes in cellular phenotype.

Studies conducted for the National Institute on Drug Abuse by Dr. Michael Iadarola and colleagues suggest that the short-term stimulus of a single dose of cocaine may cause physiological effects in the brain long after the cocaine has cleared the system.[29] Researchers found that a single dose of cocaine in rats caused an eightfold increase in c-*fos* proteins in the brain up to 24 hours after the cocaine dose. Other studies have found significant c-*fos* increases after cocaine-related seizures in rats.

The proliferation of c-*fos* proteins may help to explain how cocaine can trigger changes in the neurons' genetic expression, the redefinition of the chemical environment as normal, the number of receptors, and the powerful and long-lasting cravings and memory-like effects reported by cocaine users. Furthermore, the changes in gene expression caused by cocaine may explain the phenomenon of "kindling" as well as the high incidence of panic attacks among cocaine addicts.[30] Kindling refers to the process whereby repeated administration of cocaine may induce seizures at levels previously tolerated by the brain. Eventually, the seizures may occur even in the absence of cocaine. Even though there is no cocaine, the memory of cocaine produced through altered gene expression may be sufficient to induce seizures. Similarly, the altered gene expression may trigger a physiological reaction, classified by the user as a panic attack, even in the absence of cocaine administration.

The Effects of Varying Routes of Administration

The precise psychological and behavioral effects depend on many factors: the purity of the drug; route of administration; chronicity of use; the genetics, personality, and mental health of the user; past and present use of drugs and alcohol; the environment in which the drug is used; and other drugs taken at the same time. Table 3.4 compares cocaine's effects following different routes of administration.

The purer the drug, the greater its specific neurobiological and behavioral effects. As a rule, pure cocaine is unavailable on the street. Instead, cocaine is usually adulterated with other substances such as mannitol, lactose, or glucose to add weight, and caffeine, lidocaine, amphetamines, quinine, or even heroin to add taste and to provide additional central nervous system (CNS) stimulant effects.[31] The typical concentration of cocaine in street preparations ranges from 10 to 50%; rarely, samples can contain as much as 70% cocaine. Both the cocaine concentration and the adulterants affect the user's response to the drug. Even the accurate medical historian cannot determine whether the illicit cocaine consumed was really cocaine or caffeine and/or lidocaine, mannitol, and so on.

The Rewarding Effects of Other Drugs

Cannabis Reinforcement

Unlike other drugs of abuse, marijuana had previously been thought to lack any pharmacological interaction with the brain's reward system. However, it now appears that marijuana's principal psychoactive ingredient, delta^9-tetrahydrocannabinol (delta^9-THC), acts as a DA agonist in a manner similar to other noncannabinoid drugs of abuse.[6] In addition, delta^9-THC has been shown to bind with the distinct opioid receptor subtype called the μ receptor. Chen and colleagues have demonstrated that delta^9-THC adminis-

TABLE 3.4. Differential Effects Dependent on Routes of Cocaine Administration

Administration		Initial onset of action (sec)	Duration of "high" (min)	Average acute dose (mg)	Peak plasma levels (ng/mL)	Purity (%)	Bioavailability (percent absorbed)
Route	Mode						
Oral	Coca leaf chewing	300–600	45–90	20–50	150	0.5–1	—
Oral	Cocaine HCl	600–1800	—	100–200	150–200	20–80	20–30
Intranasal	"Snorting" cocaine HCl	120–180	30–45	5 × 30	150	20–80	20–30
Intravenous	Cocaine HCl	30–45	10–20	25–50 >200	300–400 1000–1500	7–100 × 58	100
Smoking	Coca paste	8–10	5–10	60–250	300–800	40–85	6–32
Intrapulmonary	Freebase crack	—	—	250–1000	800–900 ?	90–100 50–95	—

SOURCE: Gold, MS. *800 Cocaine.* New York: Bantam Books, 1985. Reprinted with permission.

tration enhances presynaptic DA levels at brain reward loci[32] and that this increase can be attenuated by the opiate antagonist naloxone.[33] Naloxone's alteration of delta[9]-THC effects suggests that marijuana engages endogenous brain opioid circuitry and formulates an essential association between these endogenous opioids and DA neurons in the MFB. Furthermore, this association appears fundamental to marijuana's positive effects on the brain's reward system and, ultimately, marijuana's abuse potential.

Opiate Reinforcement

Although the primary opiate effect is sedation mediated by μ opioid receptors, opiates have been shown to provoke the dopaminergic cells of the ventral tegmental area and the substantia nigra, sometimes to the point of exhaustion.[34] As with marijuana, opiate ability to engage endogenous opiate receptors may be associated with the increased DA activity. Opiates produce their analgesia, respiratory depression, hypotension, and axiolytic effects by binding with the δ (delta) and μ-receptors and inhibiting adenylate cyclase. This inhibition results in diminished conversion of adenosine triphosphate (ATP) to cyclic adenosine monophosphate (cAMP) and decreased phosphoprotein levels. It has been suggested that opiate withdrawal may result in a rebound increase in cAMP levels.[35]

Studies showing that direct injections of opiates into the ventral tegmental area activate feeding and provide additional support for the role of opiate interaction with the DA system in the reward process.[36,37] In addition, pharmacological inhibition of the DA sys-

tem in hungry and thirsty animals reduces the reinforcing effects of food and water.[38]

Gardner and others have found that the brain
reward enhancement produced by drugs of abuse
like opiates, cocaine, amphetamines, ethanol, and benzodiazepines is attenuated by opiate antagonists like
naloxone and naltrexone.[39] Naloxone-induced attenuation of BSR created by all known classes of abusable
drugs supports the importance of endogenous opioid
systems in all drugs of abuse and not just opioids.
The opioid-dopamine connections are now the focus
of scientific study to explain the abuse of all drugs
and alcohol.

Neuroanatomical study supports the interrelation-
ship between dopamine and opioid systems, since cell
bodies, axons, and synaptic terminals of enkephalin-
containing and endorphinergic neurons are found
throughout the extent of the mesotelencephalic dopamine axon terminals, forming an axo-axonic synapse
that could modulate the flow of dopamine and the
reward signals through the existing and well-described
dopamine circuitry. Some dopamine reward neurons
may synapse directly on opioid peptide neurons.

Nicotine has also been found to enhance DA levels
and to be a positive reinforcer, although not to the
same extent as cocaine. DA release in the nucleus accumbens has occurred in vitro in response to small
concentrations of nicotine.[40] This DA effect of nicotine
may explain the addictive power of tobacco.

Factors other than pharmacological effects of abused
drugs may lead to positive reinforcement. For example,
drug use may be viewed positively by a subculture
and thereby enhance a user's social standing, encour-

age approval by drug-using friends, and convey a special status to the user.

Learning as an Outcome of Reinforcement

As demonstrated above, cocaine and opiates, on a basic or primitive level, produce rapid reinforcement described as a drug "high" or "rush." This reward is clearly neurobiological in that the drug use stimulates its own taking and produces a sense of organismic accomplishment similar to species-specific survival behaviors. Drug users feel as if they have acted to preserve the species, when in reality they have simply bypassed the normal behavior reward system.

Drug use provides a quick and powerful means of changing one's moods and sensations. In a cost-to-benefit analysis, the user seeks the immediately gratifying effects as a "benefit" that outweighs the long-term adverse cost of drug use. Other users may be influenced by physical or psychological states such as depression, pain, or stress that may be temporarily relieved by drug consumption. Drug use is such a powerful reinforcer and shaper of behavior that drug paraphernalia and virtually all of the sights, smells, and events associated with finding and using drugs become reinforcers.

The changes in mood associated with drug reinforcement serve as an unconditioned stimulus. Given frequent association with these changes, a variety of other factors, including the psychological (mood states, cognitive expectations of euphoria, stress, and so on) and environmental (drug paraphernalia, drug-using locations or friends, and so on), can become conditioned stimuli in a manner similar to the classic Pavlov canine experiments. Exposure to these cocaine-conditioned stimuli can precipitate the "taste" of the drug, leading to intense drug craving and withdrawal-like physiological responses that the user interprets as drug cravings and that often lead to relapse.[41] (For more information on craving and conditioned relapse, see the discussion with Dr. Charles O'Brien on pp. 57–60.)

Animal studies demonstrating a conditioned place preference (CPP) for cocaine show how environment can be associated with drug use. In these studies, an animal receives either a saline or a cocaine-containing solution and then is confined to one side of a chamber. Later, the drug-free animal is allowed to roam freely throughout the chamber while time spent in either side is recorded. The animals soon show a distinct preference for the side associated with the cocaine injection. Interestingly, administration of the mixed opioid agonist-antagonist buprenorphine has recently been shown to attenuate cocaine CPP, again suggesting the involvement of the opioid system in cocaine-related reward.[42]

Withdrawal

While significant evidence supports the role of dopamine in the reward process, the neuroanatomy of withdrawal, apparently anatomically distinct from the reward system, is not as clearly defined. However, a wide variety of abused drugs, with apparently little in common pharmacologically, share common withdrawal effects (see Table 3.5, p. 61) associated with the locus coeruleus (LC).

Support for a shared withdrawal pathway also stems from similarities in withdrawal treatment—opi-

Conditioned Responses, Craving, Relapse and Addiction:
A Discussion with Charles P. O'Brien, M.D., Ph.D.,
Professor and Vice Chairman, Department of Psychiatry,
University of Pennsylvania and Chief of Psychiatry,
VA Medical Center

Q: *Can you explain why relapse is the rule rather than the exception in addiction?*

A: The concept of relapse is very hard for the general public to understand. To them relapse is failure. I try to stress that it is not really failure and that they should see addiction as a chronic disorder. Think of someone being treated for depression: the patient may leave the hospital with antidepressant medication. Now they still have days when they feel depressed—the symptoms don't completely go away. But these brief periods of feeling depressed do not mean that their treatment is failed. Overall, the syndrome is so much better that they are able to go back to work. We need to look at addiction the same way.

But the public considers a person having one drink or one shot of heroin to have immediately relapsed and it is not so—even if they have a binge. If they return to treatment, go back to remission, then their treatment hasn't failed. While you certainly don't want to encourage these slips, you have to recognize it as a slip, a slip that can be studied with a patient to uncover why it occurred. Perhaps the most important point is that the public should understand that relapse can be contained, and that it does not automatically mean a return to addiction.

Q: *What causes a person to "slip"?*

A: There are many possible causes. One possible cause that we have studied intensively is the conditioned response. Basically a conditioned response is a learned association between a stimulus that has been neutral, such as a smell or sound of a bell that doesn't mean anything to the subject, and something that has a reflexive effect, such as food that automatically makes a person salivate or a drug that produces an effect.

(continued)

After repeated pairings of the neutral stimulus and the drug effect, the neutral stimulus acquires the ability to produce the drug effect. That's called a conditioned response. There are some exciting basic studies that suggest these conditioned response result in memory traces that are stored in the brain.

Q: *What is the connection between a conditioned response and craving for a drug?*
A: Well, first you have to define craving. Craving can only be measured by subjective effects—by what people tell us—and they tell us that they feel a sudden, strong desire for drugs.

Our studies have shown, and other people have reported as well, that certain things make an addict crave. For alcoholics it may be simply passing a bar, or smelling alcohol; for cocaine addicts it may be seeing someone using cocaine. These become triggers, or conditioned cues, that provoke craving. We think that this occurs because there has previously been an association in the use of this drug and this stimulus, whatever it happens to be. In fact for cocaine it can be very dramatic— some experienced users tell us that they start feeling "high" *before* they actually take the cocaine into their body.

What we think might be going on is that there is a conditioned response that produces an increase in dopamine in the area of the brain called the nucleus accumbens. Animal studies using microdialysis show an increase in dopamine levels in the nucleus accumbens every time the animal gets cocaine. An interesting phenomenon occurs when saline is administered after several days of cocaine. The animal still thinks they are going to get cocaine and their dopamine levels increase even though they are only getting saline. Effectively, the conditioned response is like a "mini-dose" of cocaine, sometimes called a "priming dose." A small priming dose tends to provoke more desire for the drug.

Q: *Why do some effective medications used to treat cocaine addiction, such as amantadine or bromocriptine, also cause increases in functional dopamine activity?*
A: We have data that show that amantadine helps addicts to achieve abstinence. Since amantadine increases dopaminergic function it is analogous to giving a low dose of an opiate to an

opiate addict who is in withdrawal—you're basically giving them a small amount of what they had previously gotten in large amounts and this reduces their withdrawal. However if they are over their withdrawal, completely drug-free, and then you give them this low dose you would be giving them a "priming dose" that increases the risk of relapse. The same thing that helps withdrawal can also hasten relapse when given at another time.

Q: *Could you describe some of your work with provoked craving?*
A: We have been studying the responses of cocaine addicts to videos of people using cocaine. We have found that these videos are very strong at provoking craving and also at provoking arousal. This arousal is measured by increases in blood pressure and heart rate, and by decreases in skin temperature and skin resistance. Basically when they simply view a video, they get an arousal response that is very much like taking cocaine or another stimulant.

Q: *Are these physical responses associated with verbal acknowledgment of their craving?*
A: That's an interesting question because they are often correlated: the person feels high and admits they want more. However, some patients deny that they are feeling anything even though their polygraph shows them going off the chart. And there are some people who say they experience the craving but we don't see anything on their polygraph. So we can't say that there is a perfect correlation by any means.

Q: *Are there any data on which of the two groups has the higher relapse rate?*
A: We just presented some preliminary data that show that those people with the strong physical reaction to the cocaine cues have a higher relapse rate—the stronger the reaction the higher the relapse rate.

Q: *How do you explain why many addicts who relapse in treatment indicate other factors, such as boredom and depression, and not craving as the reason for their relapse?*
A: It may be that they are not even aware of their craving on
(continued)

a conscious level and that they really don't understand why they relapse. They may simply see a drug-using friend and before they know it, their behaviorally conditioned response has taken over and they have relapsed to drug use. Of course, as I stated at the beginning, there are many reasons for relapse and we have to pay attention to all of them, not just conditioning.

Q: *Is craving related to relapse?*
A: It's a complex question because a person can feel craving and not give in to it. Just because they crave doesn't mean that they have to relapse and so I think you will always find a mixed response to this question. Some people don't like the term craving at all because it means different things to different people. But it seems to have operational value: we can use it with patients and they can rate craving and they can do it in a systematic way.

Q: *What should be the goal of addiction treatment?*
A: Perhaps the most important point to remember is that addiction is a chronic disorder. When a patient goes into remission through detoxification, they are not really over that disorder any more than anyone with heart disease or arthritis is cured when their pain stops. For addicts, it could very well be that the conditioned response, the memory trace, is still there waiting to reactivate the addictive behavior under the right circumstances. It is very difficult to treat.

But the goal of addiction treatment should not be limited to abstinence because that is very elusive and difficult to achieve. Since addiction is a chronic disorder you should aim to have patients with longer periods of abstinence, longer remissions. It may be difficult to the public to accept, but if recovering addicts are only using drugs occasionally where before they were using every day—that's progress.

Source: Adapted with permission from MS Gold (Ed.), the University of Florida's *Facts About Drugs and Alcohol Newsletter*, 1(4), 1992.

TABLE 3.5. Withdrawal Symptoms of Abused Drugs

Alcohol	Opiates	Benzodiazepines	Tobacco	Cocaine
Nervousness	Nervousness	Nervousness	Nervousness	Nervousness
Tachycardia	Tachycardia	Bradycardia	Bradycardia	Bradycardia
Hyperpyrexia	Hyperpyrexia	Hyperpyrexia		
Insomnia	Insomnia	Insomnia		Hypersomnia
Disrupted sleep	Disrupted sleep	Disrupted sleep	Disrupted sleep	REM rebound
Irritability	Irritability	Irritability	Irritability	Irritability
Agitation	Agitation	Agitation	Agitation	Psychomotoric retardation
Restlessness	Restlessness	Restlessness	Restlessness	Restlessness
Anorexia	Anorexia	Hyperphagia	Hyperphagia	Hyperphagia
Tremor	Tremor	Tremor		
Hypertension	Hypertension			
Hyperarousal	Hyperarousal	Hyperarousal	Impatience	Hypoarousal
Sweating	Sweating			
Nausea and vomiting	Nausea and vomiting			
Fear	Fear	Fear		
Craving	Craving	Craving	Craving	Craving
	Lacrimation, rhinorrhea, gooseflesh, pain			
	Spontaneous orgasm, yawning			
Depression	Depression	Depression		Depression

ates, nicotine, benzodiazepines, and alcohol have all had their withdrawal symptoms treated effectively by clonidine, a medication that suppresses LC hyperactivity.

Gawin and Kleber have identified a three-stage pattern that often develops following abstinence from cocaine use.[43] The first stage is the immediate cocaine "crash" similar to an alcoholic hangover and characterized by low energy, depression, bradykinesis, weight gain, and hypersomnia. The hypersomnia may last several days before mood stabilization occurs.

From 0.5 to 4 days after the first stage comes the second, or withdrawal, phase, with continuing depression, anhedonia, anxiety, lack of motivation, fatigue, and sleep disturbance. This anhedonic state contrasts markedly with the user's memories of cocaine-induced euphoria and may trigger cocaine cravings that lead to renewed cocaine consumption. This withdrawal phase correlates to elements of the withdrawal states found in other drugs of abuse. (Anxiety is the hallmark of opiate, nicotine, alcohol, and sedative/hypnotic withdrawal, while anhedonia and sleep disturbances are common to all—see Table 3.5.) Cocaine abstinence is generally devoid of overtly "catastrophic" physical symptoms. The delirium tremens or withdrawal seizures associated with benzodiazepines, alcohol, and sedative/hypnotic withdrawal, and the nausea and vomiting associated with opiate withdrawal, are usually not associated with cocaine withdrawal. In the past, awareness of the reality of cocaine dependence has been limited primarily because of the subtlety of its abstinence symptoms and the belief that physical withdrawal is necessary.

Cocaine users, aware of the dangers of continued

use and motivated to remain abstinent or in treatment, may be able to endure this anhedonic period if not confronted by a powerful conditioned cue. (Perhaps the primary benefit of inpatient treatment is the patient's removal from the drug-using environment and from access to illegal drugs.) Cocaine and amphetamines are the most potent drug reinforcing agents known, and use of these agents results in profound classical and operant conditioning.[44] The conditioned cue will often ignite an intense craving for cocaine that combines with the anhedonic craving to present the patient with a formidable obstacle to recovery. A conditioned cue may occur after interaction with a "person, place, or thing" (that is, locations, holidays, events, drug paraphernalia) associated with previous drug use. Even positive or negative mood states may be perceived as a conditioned cue.

The third phase involves the gradual extinguishing of drug cravings. If a lasting recovery is to be achieved, abstinence must persist in the face of powerful, intermittent conditioned craving. A period ranging from a few months to several years may be necessary for the dissipation of these conditioned cravings.

The basis for the delineation of the three phases originated from clinical observation and study. Subsequently, these phases were verified in a large-scale outpatient study, although results among studies of hospitalized patients have been mixed.[43] For example, a study of inpatients by Satel and colleagues found that the symptoms of cocaine withdrawal are relatively mild and transient.[44] One explanation for this apparent discrepancy may be the lack of conditioned cues in the hospital environment. In the absence of these cues, the anhedonic period may pass with relatively little discomfort.

In addition, the relative dearth of withdrawal symptoms may explain, at least partially, the episodic patterns of use reported by many cocaine addicts where periods of intense cocaine bingeing alternate with intervals of abstinence. Because chronic cocaine administration has been shown to decrease brain levels of DA and norepinephrine (NE) while inhibiting LC activity,[45,46] one might expect that abstinence in cocaine abusers would trigger LC activity and subsequent withdrawal symptoms in a manner similar to opiate withdrawal; however, it appears that NE depletion limits the withdrawal response.[47] The intense craving and high recidivism rate associated with cocaine use appears to derive more from a nucleus accumbens withdrawal dysphoria and a drive to repeat a pleasurable experience rather than avoid the discomfort of LC withdrawal.

The Role of Craving in Relapse

While no cause for drug addiction has been found and a multiplicity of theories abound, most theories include drug craving in the etiology of addiction, the persistence of use, and the high relapse rates of addicts. Most attempts by experts to characterize drug addiction rely heavily on craving, or the overpowering urge, for the drug. Craving is invoked as the likely culprit to explain drug seeking during the height of withdrawal or to explain a "weekend" slip. The entire subject of craving has been very controversial. Even when alcohol experts discuss alcohol craving there is much disagreement. Is craving limited to the acute withdrawal period, or can it occur at any time and be evidenced by loss of control and relapse? Jellinek rejected craving in the abstinent state, as did Isbell, who argued, "After a few days or weeks of abstinence, the alcoholic . . . is physiologically indistinguishable from his fellows. He has no craving in the physical sense, yet he relapses and drinks to excess again."[48]

Dysphoric mood states, drug availability and provocation by drug stimuli appear to clinicians treating cocaine addicts to be far better predictors of relapse than either physical withdrawal or self-reports of craving. Ludwig reported that only 1% of relapsing alcoholics attributed their relapse after treatment to craving.[49] Psychological distress, family problems, and alcohol's positive effects were the most frequently cited explanations. Marlatt reported that only 5% of relapsers gave craving as the reason for relapse to alcohol and other drug urges.[50] These findings have been replicated by Littman and colleagues.[51] Similarly, only 6% of opiate relapsers listed craving as the most important factor in relapse in a recent study.[52] And Wallace reported only 5.7% of crack smokers as listing craving as the cause of their relapse.[53]

More recent studies have suggested that the best predictors of relapse were the subjects' physiological response to drug cues and not conscious responses. Kennedy, studying pupillary dilation, recently reported that persistence of pupillary dilation in the presence of the subjects' favorite alcoholic beverage predicted relapse.[54] Niaura and colleagues reported that the cardiovascular response (reduced heart rate) to a nicotine cue predicted relapse.[54,55]

As reviewed by Tiffany, motivated behaviors can occur in the absence of consciously experienced needs, urges, or cravings.[56] In our most recent report, we have shown that drug craving and relapse are independent.[57] Cocaine relapse is related by patients to "unknown" or "impulsive" actions (see Table 3.6).

Drug seeking and use are highly practiced automatic behaviors in the addict, who may not require the intervention of conscious thoughts or distinct craving states. *Craving may not be experienced at a conscious level but rather may be experienced as a physiological drive.* It is interesting that when recovering addicts complain of craving, this is a good prognostic sign. Daily treatment or Alcoholics Anonymous (AA) not only may provide support for the recovering addict and keep current the prospects and outcome of a relapse but may help the addict learn to identify craving and means of prescribing people and time to avoid a relapse. It is almost as if the unconscious craving or drive for the drug at a limbic or nucleus accumbens level results in relapse, while verbalized, cortical craving represents early and somewhat successful attempts to control this new drive.

TABLE 3.6. Cause of First Relapse

Cause of relapse (first use)	Alcohol (AD)	Drug (CD)
Craving	7%	7%
Impulsive action	11%	41%
Social pressure	9%	11%
Depressed	20%	11%
Tense	13%	11%
Happy or excited	11%	11%
Decided risks were minimal	0%	11%
Other	19%	8%

Not all craving leads to drug taking. Successful treatment may amount to making craving conscious and controllable through learning and cortical control over acquired (limbic) drive states.

Other Areas of Interest

The Nucleus Accumbens and Ventral Tegmental Area in Reward

A wide range of sites appear to moderate the brain stimulant reward of both opiates and stimulants. For example, microinjection of amphetamine into the nucleus accumbens (NAc) facilitated stimulation response in the ventral tegmental area (VTA), while morphine injections into the NAc did not enhance stimulation response in the VTA.[58] Evidence suggests that cocaine (and possibly other abused psychoactive compounds) produces its rewarding effect by increasing synaptic DA concentrations and consequently producing a critical increase in the stimulation of NAc DA receptors. Thus, cocaine increases NAc DA concentrations by binding to a DA transporter and thereby inhibiting reuptake of DA into presynaptic neurons.[59] In operant conditioning experiments where animals have been shown to self-administer large quantities of cocaine and many other compounds abused by humans, the potency of various cocaine-related compounds in maintaining self-administration behavior can be predicted by each compound's affinity for the DA transporter.[60] In contrast, self-administration behavior is not predictable from drug affinities for norepinephrine or serotonin transporters.[60] Furthermore, the rewarding effects of cocaine self-administration are reduced by D_1 and D_2 receptor antagonists but not by noradrenergic receptor antagonists.[61] Finally, self-administration of cocaine is reduced or eliminated following lesions of the dopaminergic innervation of the NAc or lesions of NAc cell bodies.[62] In contrast, lesions of noradrenergic or dopaminergic terminals in the striatum or prefrontal cortex are without effect.[63]

Similar studies suggest that amphetamine produces its rewarding effects through activation of NAc DA receptors.[64] Opiate abuse may also be related to the stimulation of NAc DA receptors. However, the data are equivocal.[65,66] It is also worth noting that nicotine, tetrahydrocannabinol (THC), and alcohol increase NAc DA concentration.[32]

Finally, evidence suggests that the DA receptors of the NAc may function as part of a neuronal mechanism responsible for endogenous reward that reinforces behaviors leading to natural stimuli such as food and water. Thus, operant conditioning experiments with animals indicate that the rewarding properties of food, water, or intracranial brain stimulation may depend on the NAc DA receptor activation.[67] Therefore, the rewarding properties of drugs that lead to excessive self-administration may result from the ability of these compounds to activate this neural substrate for endogenous reward.

The Locus Coeruleus in Withdrawal

Although the locus coeruleus has been studied primarily in reference to opiate withdrawal, recent research has suggested its involvement in withdrawal from a wide range of abused drugs, including cocaine. Located in the dorsolateral pontine tegmentum of all mammals is the nucleus locus coeruleus, a densely packed cell grouping that was first described in 1809. The locus coeruleus was named for its blueish color, which derives from the presence of neuromelanin, making it a rather easily identified nucleus on cross section. With the invention of fluorescent staining techniques, this bilateral brain stem nucleus lying along the fourth ventricle beneath the cerebellar peduncles was found to contain the neurotransmitter norepinephrine. The human LC is the largest grouping of NE-containing neurons in the brain, consisting of roughly 18,000 cells and the most extensive network of pathways emanating from any nucleus in the brain. The LC is the largest nucleus of central noradrenergic neurons in the mammalian central nervous system and is the origin of virtually all noradrenergic afferents in the brain.[68] LC neurons extensively innervate many brain sites with highly branched axons. Even single LC neurons project simultaneously to different brain sites from many axonal branches. Ungerstedt has suggested that a single LC cell probably projects to the cerebrum, hippocampus, and cerebellum simultaneously, forming a tree of collateral axons.[69] Such a network gives the LC the anatomical capability to integrate the functional activity of many brain regions and influence brain function and reactivity in a very important way.

LC neurons receive sensory input from many or possibly all peripheral sensory modalities. The LC neurons have a great capacity to undergo axonal sprouting in response to environmental stimuli. When animals are exposed to repeated environmental stimuli such as stress, the LC may attain a greater capacity to affect their target neurons by increasing the density of their terminal axons.

Normally, the LC is activated by pain, blood loss, and cardiovascular collapse but not by nonthreatening stimuli.[70] However, in the opiate-dependent animal, abstinence or the administration of the opiate antagonists naloxone and naltrexone clears opiates from the μ receptor and places neurons in the LC into a state of hyperexcitability, also referred to as rebound from chronic inhibition or LC hyperactivity.[69,71] The resultant noradrenergic hyperactivity and release is an essential factor in the precipitation of withdrawal symptoms and signs.

Grant and colleagues demonstrated that behavioral patterns associated with electrical activation of the LC also occur during opiate withdrawal in nonhuman primates, thereby directly establishing that the LC hyperactivity seen during opioid withdrawal is responsible for all or a major portion of the opioid withdrawal syndrome.[72] Furthermore, other studies have confirmed that the LC cells become tolerant and dependent to opiate administration, that the cells are hyperactive during withdrawal,[73] and that the actual chronology of opiate withdrawal effects correlates with the in vivo activity of LC and increased activity in G-proteins, adenylate cyclase, and cAMP-dependent protein kinase in the rat LC.[74]

Studies showing that withdrawal activation of the LC is not observed in isolated slice preparations and by lesions of the paragigantocellularis (the major excitatory input to the LC) suggest the importance of this input to the LC hyperactivity in withdrawal.[75,76] Lesions of the glutaminergic nucleus paragigantocellu-

laris, in addition to excitatory amino acid antagonists, can suppress opiate withdrawal.[77,78] A recent
study using antagonists of the N-methyl-d-aspartate
(NMDA) subtype of excitatory amino acid receptors lessened morphine withdrawal behaviors while not apparently reversing LC hyperactivity.[79] Finally, direct
naloxone infused onto the LC leads to withdrawal
symptoms approximate to systemic naloxone spontaneous withdrawal.

   The LC may also become hyperactive in other
drug withdrawal states. Numerous states have chroni-
cled ethanol's ability to suppress LC activity,[80,81] with
significant evidence supporting the role of alpha-2 adre-
noreceptors in the pathogenesis of alcohol addiction.
An alpha-2 agonist, clonidine, has been shown to be
effective in treating alcohol withdrawal.[82] Clonidine's
efficacy in benzodiazepine, alcohol, nicotine, and opiate withdrawal supports a common LC withdrawal
hyperactivity theory.[83] Recently, administration of the
alpha-2 antagonist yohimbine has been found to re-
verse the LC inhibition of ethanol.[84] This finding and
clonidine's efficacy suggest that the alpha-2 receptors
are involved in LC inhibition, in the development of
ethanol tolerance, and even in withdrawal. Furthermore, this finding presents the possibility that a novel
morphine/yohimbine combination medication may provide effective analgesia with a decreased risk of addiction.

Clinical Implications

   LC hyperactivity may be the cause of the "physical" withdrawal syndrome for a wide variety of drugs,
but drug use clearly does not occur only to prevent

withdrawal suffering. It may be that withdrawal effects associated with the nucleus accumbens may account for the affective symptoms of withdrawal (see Table 3.1). All abuse-prone drugs are used, at least initially, for their positive effects and because the user believes the short-term benefits of this experience surpass the long-term costs. Although drug reinforcement can be eliminated by setting up a pharmacological blockade (for example, naltrexone) or by switching an inert for an active drug, the successful treatment of withdrawal is far more complicated. Studies with human opiate addicts[85,86] have shown that opiate self-administration does not occur spontaneously during naltrexone or antagonist blockade. Humans quickly identify themselves as opiate available or unavailable and change their behavior without changing their attachment to the drug and its effects. Once an antagonist is discontinued, the untreated addict continues self-administration. These data on the difficulties of lasting suppression of drug self-administration behavior are in agreement with Griffiths et al.[87]

The treatment implications of reward and withdrawal are discussed in greater detail in subsequent chapters. Before this discussion, however, a thorough presentation of the clinical manifestations of cocaine abuse is necessary.

References

1. Miller NS, Mahler JC, Belkin BM, Gold MS. Psychiatric diagnosis in alcohol and drug dependence. *Ann Clin Psychiatry.* 1990; 3 (1):79–89.
2. Grinspoon L, Bakalar JB. Chronic cocaine abuse does not usu-

ally appear as a medical problem. In: Kaplan HI, Freedman AM, Sadock BJ, eds. *Comprehensive Textbook of Psychiatry.* Baltimore, Md: Williams & Wilkins; 1980.

3. Gawin F. Cocaine addiction: psychology and neurophysiology. *Science.* March 1991; 251:1580–1586.

4. Calcagnetti DJ, Schechter MD. Conditioned place aversion following the central administration of a novel dopamine release inhibitor CGS 10746B. *Pharmacol Biochem Behav.* 1991; 40:255–259.

5. Killam KF, Olds J, Sinclair J. Further studies on the effects of centrally acting drugs on self-stimulation. *J Pharmacol Exp Ther.* 1957; 119:157.

6. Gardner EL, Lowinson JH. Marijuana's interaction with brain reward systems: update 1991. *Pharmacol Biochem Behav.* 1991; 40:571–580.

7. Crow TJ. A map of the rat mesencephalon for electrical self-stimulation. *Brain Res.* 1972; 36:265–273.

8. Wise RA, Bozarth MA. Brain substrates for reinforcement and drug self-administration. *Prog Neuropsychopharmacol.* 1981; 5:467–474.

9. Wise RA, Rompre PP. Brain dopamine and reward. *Annu Rev Psychol.* 1989; 40:191–225.

10. Dewit H, Wise RA. A blockade of cocaine reinforcement in rats with the dopamine receptor blocker pimozide but not with the noradrenergic blockers phentolamine or phenoxybenzamine. *Can J Psychol.* 1977; 31:195.

11. Wise RA. Action of drugs of abuse on brain reward systems. *Pharmacol Biochem Behav.* 1980; 13(suppl. 1):213–223.

12. Wise RA. The dopamine synapse and the notion of "pleasure centers" in the brain. *Trends Neurosci.* 1980; 3:91–95.

13. Dackis CA, Gold MS. Treatment strategies for cocaine detoxification. In: Lakoski JM, Galloway MP, White FJ, eds. *Cocaine: Pharmacology, Physiology, and Clinical Strategies.* Boca Raton, Fla: CRC Press; 1991.

14. Wise RA. The neurobiology of craving: implications for the understanding and treatment of addiction. *J Abnormal Psychol.* 1988; 97(2): 118–132.

15. Miller NS, Gold MS. The relationship of addiction, tolerance,

and dependence to alcohol and drugs: a neurochemical approach. *J Substance Abuse Treatment.* 1987;4:197–207.

16. Iverson II. *The Uptake and Storage of Noradrenaline in Sympathetic Nerves.* London: Cambridge University Press; 1967.

17. Javaid J, Fischman MW, Schuster CR, Dekirmenjian H, Davis JM. Cocaine plasma concentrations: relationship to physiological and subjective effects in humans. *Science.* 1978;202:227–228.

18. Resnick R, Schuyten-Resnick E. Clinical aspects of cocaine: assessment of cocaine abuse behavior in man. In: Mule SJ, ed. *Cocaine.* Boca Raton, Fla: CRC Press; 1977.

19. Denau GA, Yanagita T, Seevers MH. Self-administration of psychoactive substances by the monkey. *Psychopharmacologia.* 1969;16:30.

20. Pickens RL, Harris WC. Self-administration of d-amphetamine by rats. *Psychopharmacologia.* 1968;12:158.

21. Carroll FI, Lewin AH, Boja JW, Kuhar MJ. Cocaine receptor: biochemical characteristics and structure-activity relationships of cocaine analogues at the dopamine transporter. *J Medicinal Chem.* 1992;35(6):969–981.

22. Giros B, El Mestikawy S, Betrand L, Caron MG. Cloning and functional characterization of a cocaine-sensitive dopamine transporter. *FEBS Lett.* 1991;295(1,2,3):149–154.

23. Ramsey NF, van Ree JM. Intracerebroventricular naltrexone treatment attenuates acquisition of intravenous cocaine self-administration in rats. *Pharmacol Biochem Behav.* 1991;40:807–810.

24. Meert TF, Janssen PAJ. Ritanserin, a new therapeutic approach for drug abuse. Part 2: effects on cocaine. *Drug Develop Res.* 1992;25:39–53.

25. Meert TF, Janssen PAJ. Ritanserin, a new therapeutic approach for drug abuse. Part 3: effects on fentanyl and sucrose. *Drug Develop Res.* 1992;25:55–66.

26. Wolffgramm J. An ethopharmacological approach to the development of drug addiction. *Neurosci Biobehav Rev.* 1991;15:515–519.

27. Curran T, Abate C, Cohne DR, et al. Inducible proto-oncogene transcription factors: third messengers in the brain? In: *Cold Spring Harbor Symposia on Quantitative Biology.* Cold Spring Harbor Press; 1990.

28. Cohen DR, Curran T. The structure and function of the *fos* proto-oncogene. *Crit Rev Oncogen.* 1989;1:65.

29. Goodwin FK. From the Alcohol, Drug Abuse, and Mental Health Administration. *J Am Med Assoc.* December 25, 1991;266(24):3403.

30. Post R. Talk given at the American Society of Addiction Medicine's 23rd Annual Medical-Scientific Conference, April 2–5, 1992. Washington, DC.

31. Bastos ML, Hoffman DB. Detection and identification of cocaine, its metabolites and its derivatives. In: Mule SJ, ed. *Cocaine: Chemical, Biological, Clinical, Social and Treatment Aspects.* Cleveland: CRC Press; 1976:45.

32. Chen J, Paredes W, Li J, Smith D, Gardner EL. In vivo brain microdialysis studies of delta$_9$-tetrahydrocannabinol on presynaptic dopamine efflux in nucleus accumbens of the Lewis rat. *Soc Neurosci Abstr.* 1989;15:1096.

33. Chen J, Paredes W, Li J, Smith D, Lowinson J, Gardner EL. Delta$_9$-tetrahydrocannabinol produces naloxone-blockable enhancement of presynaptic dopamine efflux in nucleus accumbens of conscious, freely-moving rats as measured by intracerebral microdialysis. *Psychopharmacology* (Berlin). 1990;102:156–162.

34. Matthews RT, German DC. Electrophysiological evidence for excitation of rat ventral tegmental area dopaminergic neurons by morphine. *Neuroscience.* 1984;11:617–626.

35. Kosten TR. Neurobiology of abused drugs: opioids and stimulants. *J Nervous Mental Dis.* 1990;178(4):217–227.

36. Jenck F, Graton A, Wise RA. Opposite effects of tegmental and periaqueductal gray morphine injections on lateral hypothalamic stimulation-induced feeding. *Brain Res.* 1986;399:24–32.

37. Mucha RF, Iverson SD. Increased food intake after opioid microinjection into the nucleus accumbens and ventral tegmental area of rat. *Brain Res.* 1986;397:214–224.

38. Geary N, Smith G. Pimozide decreases the positive reinforcing effect of sham fed sucrose in the rat. *Pharmacol Biochem Behav.* 1985;22:787–790.

39. Gardner EL. Brain reward mechanism. In Lowinson JH, *Substance Abuse: A Comprehensive Textbook.* 2nd ed. Ruiz P, Millman RB, et al., eds. Baltimore, Md: Williams & Wilkins; 1992.

40. Stolerman IP, Schoaib M. The neurobiology of tobacco addiction. *Trends Pharmacol Sci.* 1991;12:467–473.

41. Winkler A. Dynamics of drug dependence: implications of a conditioning theory for research. *Arch Gen Psychiatry.* 1973;28:611–619.

42. Kosten TA, Marby DA, Nestler EJ. Cocaine conditioned place preference is attenuated by chronic buprenorphine treatment. *Life Sci.* 1991;49(24):201–206.

43. Gawin FH, Kleber HD. Abstinence symptomatology and psychiatric diagnosis in cocaine abusers: clinical observations. *Arch Gen Psychiatry.* 1986;43:107–113.

44. Satel SL, Price LH, Palumbo JM, et al. Clinical phenomenology and neurobiology of cocaine abstinence: a prospective inpatient study. *Am J Psychiatry.* 1991;148:1712–1716.

45. Dackis CA, Gold MS. Psychopharmacology of cocaine. *Psychiatric Ann.* 1988;18(9):528–530.

46. Pitts DK, Marwah J. Cocaine and central monaminergic neurotransmission: a review of electrophysiological studies and comparison to amphetamines and antidepressants. *Life Sci.* 1988;42:949–968.

47. Morton BE. The utility of viewing the locus coeruleus as an alarm system. University of Hawaii School of Medicine. In press.

48. WHO Expert Committee on Mental Health and Alcohol. The craving for alcohol. *Q J Stud Alcohol.* 1955;16:53–66.

49. Ludwig A. The mystery of craving. *Alcohol Health Res World.* 1989;11:12–17.

50. Marlatt GA. Craving for alcohol, loss of control and relapse: cognitive behavioral analysis. In: Nathan PE, Marlatt GA, Loberg T, eds. *Alcoholism: New Directions in Behavioral Research and Treatment.* New York: Plenum Press; 1978:271–314.

51. Littmen GK, Stapleton J, Oppenheim AN. Situations related to alcoholism relapse. *Br J Addict.* 1983;78:381–389.

52. Bradley BP, Phillips G, Green L, Gossop M. Circumstances surrounding the initial lapse to opiate use following detoxification. *Br J Psychiatry.* 1989;154:354–359.

53. Wallace BC. Psychological and environmental determinants of relapse in crack cocaine smokers. *J Subst Abuse Treat.* 1989;6:95–106.

54. Kennedy D. Pupillometrics as an aid in the assessment of motivation, impact of treatment and prognosis of chronic alcoholics. Unpublished doctoral dissertation. Salt Lake City: University of Utah; 1971.
55. Niaura RS, Roshenow DJ, Blinkoff JA, Monti P. Responses to smoking-related stimuli and early relapse to smoking. *Addict Behav.* 1989;14:419–428.
56. Tiffany ST. A cognitive model of drug urges and drug use behavior. *Psychol Rev.* 1990;97:147–168.
57. Gold MS, Miller NS: Dissociation of Craving and Relapse in Alcohol and Cocaine Dependence. *Soc Biol Psychiatry*, in press, 1993.
58. Juston-Lyons D, Kornetsky C. Brain-stimulation reward as a model of drug-induced euphoria: comparison of cocaine and opiates. In Lakowski J, Galloway MP, White FJ, eds. *Cocaine: Pharmacology, Physiology, and Clinical Strategies.* Boca Raton, FL: CRC Press, 1992.
59. Berger PS, Elsworth JD, Arroyo J, Roth RH. *Soc Neurosci Abstr.* 1988;14:765.
60. Ritz MC, Lamb RJ, Goldberg, Kuhar MJ. Cocaine receptors on dopamine transporters are related to self-administration of cocaine. *Science.* 1987;237:1219–1223.
61. Koob GF, Thai Le H, Creese I. The D_1 dopamine receptor antagonist SHC 23390 increases cocaine self-administration in the rat. *Neurosci Let.* 1987;79:315–320.
62. Zito KA, Vickers G, Roberts DCS. *Pharmacol Biochem Behav.* 1985;23:1029–1036.
63. Roberts DCS, Zito KA. *Methods of Assessing the Reinforcing Properties of Abused Drugs.* New York: Springer-Verlag; 1987;87–103.
64. Lyness WH, Friedle NM, Moore KE. *Pharmacol Biochem Behav.* 1979;11:553–556.
65. Pettit HO, Ettenberg A, Bloom FE, Koob GF. Destruction of dopamine in the nucleus accumbens selectively attenuates cocaine but not heroin self-administration. *Psychopharmacology.* 1984;84:167–173.
66. Nakajima S. Subtypes of dopamine receptors involved in the mechanism of reinforcement. *Neurosci Biobehav Rev.* 1989;13:123–128.
67. Stellar JR, Corbett D. Regional neuroepileptic microinjections

indicate a role for the nucleus accumbens in lateral hypothalamic self-stimulation reward. *Brain Res.* 1989;477:126–143.

68. Nakamura S, Sakaguchi T. Development and plasticity of the locus coeruleus: a review of recent physiological and pharmacological experimentation. *Prog Neurobiol.* 1990;34:505–526.

69. Gold MS, Dackis CA, Pottash ALC, et al. Naltrexone, opiate addiction and endorphins. *Med Res Rev.* 1982;2(3):211–246.

70. Amaral DG, Sinnamon HM. The locus coeruleus: neurobiology of a central noradrenergic nucleus. *Prog Neurobiol.* 1977;9:147–196.

71. Gold MS, Redmond DE Jr, Kleber HD. Clonidine in opiate withdrawal. *Lancet.* 1978;1(8070):929–930.

72. Grant SJ, Huang YH, Redmond YH. Behavior of monkeys during opiate withdrawal and locus coeruleus stimulation. *Pharmacol Biochem Behav.* 1988;30:13–19.

73. Valentino RJ, Wehby RG. Locus coeruleus discharge characteristics of morphine-dependent rats: effects of naltrexone. *Brain Res.* 1989;488:126–134.

74. Rasmussen K, Beitner-Johnson DB, Krystal JH, Aghajanian GK, Nestler EJ. Opiate withdrawal and the rat locus coeruleus: behavioral, electrophysiological and biochemical correlates. *J Neurosci.* 1990;10:2308–2317.

75. Christie MJ, Williams JT, North AR. Cellular mechanism of opioid tolerance: studies in single brain neurons. *Mol Pharmacol.* 1987; 32:633–638.

76. Rasmussen KL, Aghajanian GK. Withdrawal-induced activation of locus coeruleus neurons in opiate-dependent rats: attenuation by lesions of the nucleus paragigantocellularis. *Brain Res.* 1989;505:346–350.

77. Akaoka H, Aston-Jones G. Opiate withdrawal-induced hyperactivity of locus coeruleus neurons is substantially mediated by augmented excitatory amino acid input. *J Neurosci.* 1991; 11(12):3830–3839.

78. Tung CS, Grenhoff J, Svensson TH. Morphine withdrawal responses of rat locus coeruleus neurons are blocked by an excitatory amino acid antagonist. *Acta Physiol Scand.* 1990;138:581–582.

79. Rasmussen K, Fuller RW, Stockton ME, Perry KW, Swinford RM, Ornstein PL. NMDA receptor antagonists suppress behav-

iors but no norepinephrine turnover or locus coeruleus unit activity induced by opiate withdrawal. *Eur J Pharmacol.* 1991;197:9–16.

80. Poherecky LA, Brick J. Activity of neurons in the locus coeruleus of the rat: inhibition by ethanol. *Brain Res.* 1977;131:171–179.

81. Strahlendorf JC, Strahlendorf HK. Response of locus coeruleus neurons to direct application of ethanol. *Neurosci Abstr.* 1984;7:312.

82. Baumgartner GR, Rowen RC. Clonidine vs. chlordiazepoxide in the management of acute alcohol withdrawal syndrome. *Arch Intern Med.* 1987;147:1223–1226.

83. Gold MS, Miller NS. Seeking pleasure and avoiding pain: the neuroanatomy of reward and withdrawal. *Psychiatric Ann.* 1992;22(8):430–435.

84. Verbanck P, Seutin V, Massotte L, Dresse A. Yohimbine can induce ethanol tolerance in an in vitro preparation on rat locus coeruleus. *Alcoholism: Clin Experiment Res.* 1991;15(6):1036–1039.

85. Mello NK, Mendelson JH, Kuehnle JC, et al. Operant analysis of human heroin self-administration and the effects of naltrexone. *J Pharmacol Exp Ther.* 1980;216:45–54.

86. Meyer RE, Mirrin SV, Altman JL, et al. A behavioral paradigm for the evaluation of narcotic antagonists. *Arch Gen Psychiatry.* 1976;33:371–377.

87. Griffiths RR, Bigelow GE, Henningfield JE. Similarities in animal and human drug-taking behavior. In: Mello NK, ed. *Advances in Substance Abuse.* vol 1. Greenwich, Conn: JAI Press; 1980.

88. U. S. Department of Health and Human Services. *Alcohol and Health.* Seventh Special Report to the U. S. Congress, January 1990. DHHS Publication # (ADM) 90-1656.

89. Woolverton WL, Johnson KM. Neurobiology of cocaine abuse. *TiPs* (13):193–200. May 1992.

4

The Clinical Manifestions
of Cocaine Abuse

The clinician's task of diagnosing cocaine abuse is significantly complicated by the common tenacity of drug users in denying their drug consumption. A drug user's denial is fueled in part by the stigma society attaches to drug use and by the fact that admission of drug use threatens the continuation of the drug-using state. As a result, patient histories are a notoriously unreliable means of identifying drug use. Figure 4.1, derived from an antenatal and postpartum study of inner-city black mothers, illustrates the underreporting of contemporaneous drug use. In this study, drug use was assessed by interviews during pregnancy and 13 months after giving birth. The findings of this study that drug use during pregnancy was significantly underreported confirm other studies of different populations.[1]

The correct diagnosis of cocaine abuse is further

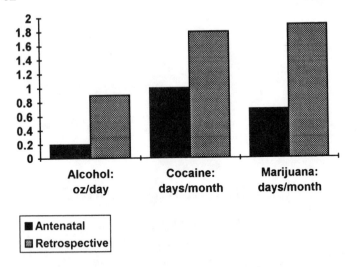

FIGURE 4.1. Alcohol and drug use by pregnant women: antenatal and retrospective reports. SOURCE: Jacobson SW, Jacobson JL, Sokol RJ, et al. Maternal recall of alcohol, cocaine, and marijuana use during pregnancy. *Neurotoxicol Teratol.* 1991;3:535–540.

complicated by the fact that patients may present with a wide range of medical and psychiatric conditions that may mask drug use. Cocaine use can adversely affect every major organ and system in the body, with cocaine-related complications including cardiovascular, respiratory, neurological, gastrointestinal, and psychiatric systems.

Acute Effects of Cocaine

Table 4.1 lists the prominent effects of a low to average dose of cocaine (approximately 20–30 mg when sniffed). These effects apply to all methods of using

TABLE 4.1. Acute Effects of Cocaine

---

1. Euphoria, seldom dysphoria
2. Increased sense of energy
3. Enhanced mental acuity
4. Increased sensory awareness (sexual, auditory, tactile, visual)
5. Decreased appetite (anorexia)
6. Increased anxiety and suspiciousness
7. Decreased need of sleep
8. Allows postponement of fatigue
9. Increased self-confidence, egocentricity
10. Delusions—dependence
11. Physical symptoms of a generalized sympathetic discharge

---

cocaine but may be more rapid and intense with cocaine smoking or intravenous (IV) use. (The different routes of administration and their acute effects are discussed in greater detail later in this chapter.)

The cocaine-induced feeling of increased alertness is reported subjectively and can be confirmed by electroencephalogram (EEG) and electrocardiogram (ECG) recordings, which show a general desynchronization of brain waves after cocaine administration.[2] Such desynchronization, which indicates arousal, occurs in the part of the brain that is thought to be involved in the regulation of conscious awareness, attention, and sleep. Despite the feeling of arousal, individuals using cocaine do not gain any particular superior ability or greater knowledge. Their sense of omnipotence is only illusional; they tend to misinterpret their enhanced confidence and lowered inhibitions as signs of enhanced physical or mental acuity.

Through its impact on the neurotransmitter system, particularly dopamine, cocaine can affect sexual excitation. Cocaine used intravenously or in smokable form can produce spontaneous ejaculation without direct genital stimulation.[3] In extreme cases cocaine even replaces the sex partner. Tolerance to the sexual stimulation of cocaine develops rapidly, sometimes resulting in impotence or sexual frigidity. Cocaine use can therefore replace the natural sex drive, which in turn threatens long-term relationships and can disrupt family stability. In some cases women cocaine users trade sexual favors for crack. During a short period of time these women may have sex with many partners, putting themselves and others at risk of infection.[4]

By inactivating the feeding center located in the lateral hypothalamus, cocaine also supersedes the primary eating drive, thus leading to severe loss of appetite and loss of body weight. Cocaine is commonly used by women with and without primary eating disorders to curb appetite or lose weight. The cocaine user's decreased need of sleep may also result from the drug's effects on neurotransmitters, including serotonin, which at times functions as the "sleep transmitter." Chronic use of the drug interferes with the ability to synthesize serotonin.

Many clinical manifestations of cocaine intoxication are also found in cases of hyperthyroidism. Some of these manifestations include hypertension, hyperkinesis, sweating, rapid heartbeat, tremor, anxiety, and hyperthermia. Conversely, the cocaine "crash" following use of the drugs shares many of the signs and symptoms with the hypothyroid state: low energy, depression, bradykinesis, weight gain, and hypersomnia. From such evidence it can be assumed that cocaine activates the thyroid axis.[5]

Dopamine acts to inhibit secretion of prolactin. By

depleting the dopamine supply, and thus robbing the body of its ability to regulate prolactin, cocaine may thus indirectly lead to hyperprolactinemia among users of the drug. Symptoms include gynecomastia, galactorrhea, and sexual dysfunctions such as infertility, impotence, and amenorrhea.

Laboratory evidence suggests that cocaine can cause adrenocortical hypertrophy, stimulating the release of high doses of cortisol in animals. It is possible that similar effects occur in humans. Thus, another aspect of cocaine use may be its impact on the hypothalamic-pituitary-adrenal (HPA) axis.[5] Because it affects the supply of acetylcholine, cocaine can lead to mental confusions and loss of coordination.[6]

Cocaine users report feeling more alert and higher in energy. This reaction in turn produces a tremendous increase in self-confidence, self-image, and egocentricity; in some individuals this manifests as megalomania and feelings of omnipotence. Some groups of people, including athletes, salespeople, entertainers, musicians, and even physicians, sometimes use cocaine to provide them with these effects, to enhance their energy and confidence.

Chronic Effects of Cocaine

There are limits to the degree that central nervous system activity can be artificially stimulated. After chronic use, or following a prolonged binge, symptoms of depression, lack of motivation, sleeplessness, paranoia, irritability, and outright acute toxic psychosis may develop.[7] States of severe transient panic accompanied by a terror of impending death can occur in persons with no preexisting psychopathological conditions, as can paranoid psychoses.[8-10]

The tremendous desire to repeat the pleasurable aspects of the cocaine experience and to counteract the depressive effects of the postcocaine crash can lead to compulsive chronic use of the drug. Such activity leads to a decrease or depletion in the neurotransmitter supply. The long-term results of such depletion include overt depression, dysphoria, hallucinatory experiences, and destructive antisocial behavior. More subtle changes in behavior include irritability, hypervigilance, psychomotor agitation, and impaired interpersonal relations.[7]

Cocaine is known to worsen the symptomatology of depression. People with biological depression are likely to experience dysphoria after cocaine use, although in other individuals cocaine acts in some ways like an antidepressant. Paranoia is another commonly seen product of cocaine abuse. In its ability to induce a state resembling functional paranoid psychosis, cocaine is similar to other central stimulants, including amphetamines.[11]

Use of cocaine can also produce a psychotic syndrome characterized by paranoia, impaired reality testing, anxiety, a stereotyped compulsive repetitive pattern of behavior, and vivid visual, auditory, and tactile hallucinations such as the delusion that insects are crawling under the skin.[11] There are also subjective and clinical data showing that cocaine can induce panic attacks.[12]

A further complication of cocaine abuse is that many users ameliorate some of the unpleasant stimulating effects of the drug by concomitantly or subsequently ingesting sedating agents, such as alcohol or marijuana.[8,13] Autopsies revealed that from 1984 to 1987, 56% of all drivers killed in traffic accidents in New York City were found to have used either cocaine, alcohol, or both.[14]

So strong is the sense of euphoria during a cocaine binge that it creates vivid, long-term memories of being high. These memories tend to persecute the drug abuser by invoking powerful cravings for the next high.[8] As will be discussed in the section on treatment, these cravings make it difficult to wean addicts from cocaine.

Medical Complications of Cocaine Abuse

The medical and psychiatric complications associated with cocaine use are so numerous and severe that it would take an entire book to describe them completely. Complications include cardiovascular effects, including arrhythmias and myocardial infarctions; respiratory effects such as chest pain and respiratory failure; neurological effects such as seizure and headache; gastrointestinal complications, including abdominal pain and nausea; and many others (see Table 4.2). For purposes of this chapter, a brief description of cocaine's far-ranging and troubling medical consequences must suffice.

Cardiovascular Complications

The first clinical report of cardiac toxicity associated with cocaine abuse appeared in 1978.[16] A review of the recent medical literature reveals that cocaine use has been linked to virtually every type of heart disease.[17]

TABLE 4.2. Medical Complications of Cocaine Abuse[15]

Cardiovascular	*Muscle*
Myocardial infarction	Rhabdomyolysis
Arrhythmia	Muscle and skin infarction
Aortic rupture	*Psychiatric*
Hypertension	Psychosis
Cardiomyopathy	Depression
Neurological	Personality changes
Stroke	Anxiety disorders
Subarachnoid hemorrhage	Delusions of parasitosis
Seizures	*Miscellaneous*
Fungal cerebritis	Acute hepatic necrosis
Dystonic reactions	Hyperpyrexia
Headache	Thrombocytopenia
Pulmonary	Loss of sense of smell
Decreased diffusing capacity	Perforated nasal septum
Pneumomediastinum	Loss of eyebrows, eyelashes
Pulmonary edema	Sexual dysfunction
Gastrointestinal	Motor vehicle accidents
Intestinal ischemia	Trauma
Colitis	Sudden death
	Endocarditis
	HIV infection

Cocaine produces a number of cardiovascular effects that may lead to the development of different forms of arrhythmia. Tachycardia often occurs within minutes of cocaine ingestion. Other forms of arrhythmia associated with cocaine use include sinus bradycardia, ventricular premature depolarization, ventricular tachycardia degenerating to defibrillation, and asystole. Crumb and Clarkson[18] suggest that cocaine may induce arrhythmias because it slows impulse conduction by blocking cardiac sodium channels. Tachycardia is also partly due to its local anesthetic activity and to indirect stimulation of alpha-receptors.[19] One study found a greater acceleration in heart rate and blood pressure associated with cocaine smoking than with intravenous cocaine use.[20]

A recent study has found a link between chronic cocaine abuse and left ventricular hypertrophy (LVH). LVH has been associated with an increased risk of arrhythmias, sudden death, and strokes. The study originated after researchers noted that several cocaine overdose victims had enlarged left ventricles without a prior history of LVH. A comparison of 30 cocaine abusers with 30 nondrug users by echocardiography revealed that the cocaine abusers had the enlarged hearts and thickened cardiac muscle associated with LVH. The hypertension associated with cocaine use may be responsible for LVH.

Cocaine is known to elevate blood pressure through adrenergic stimulation. The pressor effects of cocaine continue to rise as dosage increases.[21] The sudden increase in blood pressure may cause spontaneous bleeding in people with normal blood pressure and may underlie many incidents of cerebrovascular accidents associated with cocaine use.[22] Cerebral vasculitis has also been associated with cocaine abuse.[23]

Evidence suggests that cocaine can induce spasms in a number of vascular systems, including the coronary arteries.[24] These spasms can produce myocardial infarction even in a person whose endothelium is otherwise intact.[25] Most of the case reports of cocaine-related cardiovascular toxicity involve myocardial infarctions, which may occur regardless of dosage level or route of administration.[26] One study found a myocardial infarction rate of 31% for patients hospitalized because of cocaine-related chest pain.[27] Cocaine increases myocardial oxygen consumption, but at the same time it interferes with the coronary circulation's ability to adjust to this increased demand by decreasing its resistance to blood flow.[28] Cocaine users also frequently develop silent myocardial ischemia.[29] This problem may also arise during the first weeks of withdrawal. So common is the incidence of myocardial infarction due to cocaine that its occurrence in young patients who lack the usual coronary risk factors suggests a diagnosis of cocaine abuse.[30]

For unknown reasons, cocaine addiction can accelerate coronary atherosclerosis. Cocaine use by patients with premature artery disease can exacerbate the problem and may result in death.[31] Either directly or indirectly, cocaine may affect platelets, possibly causing them to form thrombi that can plug small vessels.[32] Finally, long-term abuse of cocaine may lead to interstitial fibrosis and eventually to congestive heart failure.[33] The cardiac effects of cocaine have previously been treated with propranolol and may respond to the calcium channel blocker nitrendipine.[5]

Respiratory Complications

Smoking crack can induce severe chest pain or dyspnea.[34] One explanation for this effect may be that cocaine significantly reduces the ability of the lungs to diffuse carbon monoxide.[35] Often it is this symptom of chest pain that drives patients to seek medical attention.

Other respiratory effects of cocaine smoking include lung damage, pneumonia, pulmonary edema, cough, sputum production, fever, hemoptysis, pulmonary barotrauma, pneumomediastinum, pneumo-thorax, pneumopericardium, and diffuse alveolar hem-orrhage.[36-38] Cocaine inhalation can cause or contribute to asthma.[39] Respiratory failure, resulting from cocaine-induced inhibition of medullary centers in the brain, may lead to sudden death.[40]

In the 1980s, a new syndrome entered the medical terminology: "crack lung."[41] People with this condition present with the symptoms of pneumonia—severe chest pains, breathing problems, and high temperatures. Yet X-rays reveal no evidence of pneumonia, and the condition does not respond to standard treatments. Anti-inflammatory drugs may relieve symptoms of crack lung. People with this syndrome may suffer oxygen starvation or loss of blood with potentially fatal results.

Neurotoxic Effects

As even Freud was aware, cocaine is an epilepto-genic agent that can provoke generalized seizures, even after a single dose.[42,43] With repeated administration, the ability of cocaine to produce chronic convulsions increases.[44] This phenomenon, known as "kindling," may result from sensitization of receptors in the brain. Repeated use of cocaine may induce chemical and elec-trical changes that, given enough time and repetition, appear to lower the brain's activity threshold. Levels of stimulation that had previously been tolerated now force an electrical discharge. Eventually this kindling reaction may occur even in the absence of cocaine and be another hidden cause of an episode of intense co-caine craving that may lead to relapse. Because seizure disorders can be unmasked or induced by cocaine's kindling effect on the brain, proper medical evaluation of patients must rule out epilepsy.[5]

As noted, cocaine abuse is associated with intracranial hemorrhage. Central nervous system stimulants such as cocaine may also cause tics; persistent, mechanical repetition of speech or movement; ataxia; and disturbed gait, which may disappear after drug use is stopped.[45]

Impact on Sexuality

Many users claim cocaine is an aphrodisiac. Indeed, as mentioned previously, the feeling of sexual excitement that sometimes accompanies cocaine use may be the result of its impact on the dopamine system and may produce spontaneous orgasm. Nonetheless, chronic cocaine abuse causes derangements in reproductive function including impotence and gynecomastia.[46] These symptoms may persist for long periods of time, even after use of cocaine has stopped. Men who abuse cocaine chronically and in high doses may have difficulty maintaining an erection and ejaculating. Many men report experiencing periods of time when they completely lose interest in sex[47]—not surprising, perhaps, given the direct effects of cocaine on the primary reward systems of the brain.

In women, cocaine abuse has adverse effects on reproductive function, including derangements in the menstrual cycle function, galactorrhea, amenorrhea, and infertility.[47] Some women who use cocaine report having greater difficulty achieving orgasm.[48] Children born to women who use cocaine during pregnancy are at high rick of congenital malformations and perinatal mortality.[49] More details on this problem appear below.

Cocaine and AIDS

Needle sharing among intravenous (IV) drug users contributes to a higher risk of human immunodefiency virus (HIV) infection and acquired immunodeficiency syndrome (AIDS) in this population and their sexual partners. As of September 1989, there were 21,188 reported cases of HIV infection in intravenous drug users, which amounted to 21% of all AIDS cases in the United States. Among the 9724 women who had been diagnosed with AIDS by September 1989, 51% of them were intravenous drug users, and an additional 19% were sexual partners of intravenous drug users. Of the 1859 children diagnosed with AIDS, 58% had mothers who used drugs intravenously or were sexual partners of intravenous drug users.[50]

Although the majority of these drug users abuse heroin, there has been a recent increase in intravenous cocaine use. The combination of cocaine use and AIDS poses two problems: First, studies indicate that cocaine may suppress the human immune system and thereby weaken the body's response to the opportunistic infections that may accompany HIV infection. Second, cocaine abuse can produce psychiatric and neurological symptoms such as depression, panic attacks, anorexia, rapid heart beats, seizures, hallucinations, and insomnia that are also associated with AIDS. The appearance of these symptoms may impede the early identification of HIV infection.

Other Adverse Effects

Chronic cocaine abuse may induce persistent hyperprolactinemia apparently because it disrupts dopamine's ability to inhibit prolactin secretion.[51] This effect may continue for long periods even after a person has stopped using cocaine.[5]

As a result of the drug's effects on the primary eating drive, many individuals who use cocaine compulsively lose their appetites and can experience significant weight loss.[52] Chapter 9 discusses eating disorders and cocaine in greater detail.

Cocaine has also been shown to produce hyperpyrexia, or extremely elevated body temperatures,[53] which can contribute to the development of seizures, life-threatening cardiac arrhythmias, and death.[54,55] This effect results from hypermetabolism combined with severe peripheral vasoconstriction and the impact of cocaine on the ability of the thalamus to regulate body heat.[56] Experimental evidence suggests that treatment for hyperpyrexia may involve vigorous cooling of the body by immersing the trunk and the extremities in cold water.[57]

Several investigators implicate cocaine in the development of the muscle-wasting condition known as rhabdomyolysis.[58,59] Why the drug should produce this effect is unclear. Roth and colleagues suggest it may arise because of arterial vasoconstriction, which can lead to tissue ischemia, or it may be due to a direct toxic effect of cocaine on muscle metabolism.[60] A study of 39 patients with acute rhabdomyolysis found that onset was rapid and occurred in previously healthy individuals who used cocaine hydrochloride. A third of this group had acute renal failure, often together with several hepatic dysfunctions and disseminated intravascular coagulation. Seven patients became oliguric, and eight required hemodialysis. Six of the 13 patients with acute renal failure died, adding yet another fatal side effect to cocaine's already long list. It has been suggested that toxicological evidence of cocaine should be sought in unexplained cases of rhabdomyolysis.[61]

Different routes of cocaine administration can produce different adverse effects. Intranasal use can lead to loss of the sense of smell, atrophy of the nasal mucosa, nose bleeds, perforation of the nasal septum, problems swallowing, and hoarseness.[62,63] Ingested cocaine can cause severe bowel ischemia or gangrene due to vasoconstriction and reduced blood flow.[64] Intravenous use is associated with diseases introduced by dirty needles contaminated with the blood of previous users as well as with extra substances in the drug (see Table 4.3). The most common severe complications from IV cocaine use are bacterial or viral endocarditis, hepatitis, and AIDS.[65] Other conditions arising from intravenous cocaine use include cellulitis, cerebritis, wound abscess, sepsis, arterial thrombosis, renal infarction, and thrombophlebitis. As mentioned previously, crack smoking can lead to the pneumonialike symptoms of crack lung. Deaths have occurred from all forms of cocaine administration.[66,67]

Other medical complications include headache, thallium poisoning, retinal artery occlusion, dermatological problems, and muscle and skin infarction. There is also a case report of a possible association between cocaine and scleroderma in a young black male.[68] Persons who

TABLE 4.3. Medical Complications of Parental Drug Use[15]

Infections	Pulmonary
Infective endocarditis	Pulmonary edema
Pneumonia	Pneumothorax
Cellulitis	Pneumomediastinum
Cutaneous abscess	Pulmonary fibrosis
Gas gangrene	Pulmonary hypertension
Infected false aneurysm	Gastrointestinal
Osteomyelitis	Motility disorders
Septic arthritis	Constipation
Sexually transmitted disease	Neuromuscular
Tuberculosis	Stroke
Tetanus	Epidural abscess
Malaria	Subdural abscess
HIV infection	Brain abscess
HTLV-I/HTLV-II infection	Transverse myelitis
Hepatic	Anoxic encephalopathy
Hepatitis A, B, C, D	Peripheral neuropathy
Acute hepatitis	Horner's syndrome
Fulminant hepatic failure	Myositis
Chronic hepatitis	Miscellaneous
Cirrhosis	Overdose
Renal	Allergic reaction
Nephrotic syndrome	Pyrogenic reaction
Glomerulonephritis	Trauma
Renal failure	Needle embolus
Cardiovascular	Necrotizing angiitis
Arrhythmia	Amenorrhea
Mycotic aneurysm	Hormonal abnormalities
Thrombophlebitis	Thrombocytopenia

lack the enzyme pseudocholinesterase are at risk for sudden death from cocaine use because the enzyme is essential for metabolizing the drug. Derlet and Albertson found that 9.5% of patients attempted suicide with cocaine or as a result of cocaine intoxication.[69]

Cocaine and Pregnancy

One of the most troubling aspects of cocaine abuse is its use by pregnant women. A 1991 study estimated the yearly inpatient hospital costs of treating infants exposed to cocaine to be an astounding $500 million. In California, infants exposed to drugs (primarily cocaine) stay an average of 9 days in the hospital (compared to 2 days for normal children) and cost 13 times more ($6900 versus $522). A 1990 study conducted by Chasnoff et al. of 36 hospitals throughout the country found that 11% of women in the hospital obstetrics units had used an illegal drug during their pregnancy.[70] Statewide urine testing of women of childbearing age visiting public health clinics in Alabama found that 11.0% of all pregnant women and 15.6% of nonpregnant women tested positive for illegal drugs.[71] In this survey, overall drug use by white women was almost 50% greater than among black women (see Figure 4.2).

While the majority of information regarding cocaine and pregnancy concerns maternal drug use, a 1991 study found that cocaine use by fathers may place future offspring at risk. In this study, cocaine attached itself to the sperm prior to the sperm entering the egg.

Drug abuse during pregnancy puts two lives at risk. Pregnancy increases a woman's susceptibility to the toxic cardiovascular effects of cocaine.[72] Placental abruption, or premature separation of a normally implanted placenta, occurs in approximately 1% of pregnancies in women who use cocaine, making the drug a significant cause of maternal morbidity as well as fetal mortality.[73] Women who use cocaine during pregnancy

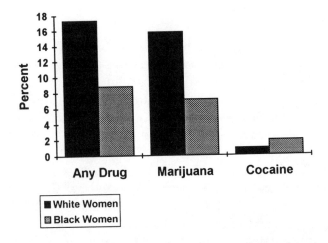

FIGURE 4.2. Statewide drug use by women of child-bearing age, by race. SOURCE: George SK, Price J, Hauth J, Barnette DM, Preston P. Drug abuse screening of childbearing-age women in Alabama public health clinics. *Am J Obstet Gynecol.* 1991;165:24–937.

have a rate of spontaneous abortion even higher than that of heroin users.

Cocaine produces toxic effects on the fetus at concentrations that are apparently nontoxic to the mother. The drug decreases blood flow to the uterus, increases uterine vascular resistance, and reduces fetal oxygen levels. The vasoconstriction, tachycardia, and increased blood pressure associated with cocaine use increase the risk of intermittent intrauterine hypoxia, preterm or precipitous labor, and placental abruption.[74] Cocaine has a significant effect on the ability of fetal hearts to produce action potentials of normal rising velocity, amplitude, and duration.[75] Maternal cocaine use has been found to affect fetal heart rate tracings, possibly because of alterations in fetal central nervous system neurotransmitters and fetal state regulation.[76] Cocaine can cause fetal cerebral infarction,[49] growth retardation,[77] and fetal death.[78]

In some parts of the country, between 15 and 25% of babies are born with cocaine already in their system.[79] The syndrome associated with cocaine-addicted infants has been named "jittery baby."[77] In one series, 34 of 39 infants exposed to cocaine before birth displayed central nervous system irritability.[80] Such children frequently present with such abnormalities as decreased birth weight, length, and head circumference; genitourinary malformations; and neurological and behavioral impairments.[49,81,82]

Chasnoff and colleagues recently reported on a 2-year follow-up growth and development outcome for three groups of infants: infants exposed to cocaine and/or other drugs during fetal development; infants exposed to marijuana and/or alcohol (but not cocaine); and infants exposed to no drugs during pregnancy.[70] Infants exposed to cocaine demonstrated significant decreases in birth weight, length, and head circumference at birth, but by 1 year of age the differences in length and weight had disappeared. However, exposure to cocaine was found to be the best predictor of head circumference. Head growth after birth may prove to be an important biological marker in predicting long-term development in children exposed in utero to cocaine.

Another recent study of drug use by pregnant women found that cocaine use was independently associated with mild facial dysmorphic features of hypertelorism and midfacial flattening in the offspring.[83] Infants of substance-abusing mothers often have a decreased ventilatory response to carbon dioxide and a 5 to 10 times increased risk of sudden infant death syndrome (SIDS).[84] Chasnoff reports that the incidence of SIDS in infants exposed to cocaine is 15%—more than three times that of infants exposed to heroin or methadone.[85] Cocaine can be passed to infants through breast milk and can be found in milk up to 60 hours after the mother used the drug. Infants intoxicated by cocaine ingested via breast milk may present with hypertension, tachycardia, sweating, dilation of the pupils, and apnea.[86] Furthermore, an emergency room study of infants and children in Detroit found that 5% tested positive for the cocaine metabolite, apparently the result of secondhand exposure to crack smoking.[87]

The effects of the drug can persist long after the child is born. Cocaine babies who survive are likely to experience visual impairments, mental retardation, and symptoms of stroke.[88] The neurological damage suffered in the womb can be permanent and can affect the child's ability to learn to function. Crack has created a new generation of people who suffer debilitating problems even before they are born.

Cocaine and Other Psychiatric Disorders

Although the exact relationship between cocaine and depression is not known, we do know that cocaine does not act as an antidepressant. Many clinicians report that cessation of cocaine use almost always alleviates the psychiatric symptoms. However, with national data showing that 76% of cocaine users have major psychiatric problems, there is still the possibility that a patient who suffers from a psychiatric illness, especially mood disorders, may be more susceptible to stimulant abuse.

Mood Disorders

Some people with depression may experiment with cocaine, amphetamines, or even excessive caffeine and tobacco in a vain attempt to lift themselves out of their fatigue, low energy, and disinterest in activities. They generally find that cocaine makes them no better and that sometimes it makes them even more depressed and hopeless. Surveys of people undergoing treatment for cocaine abuse reveal that perhaps half of a given patient population meet the diagnostic criteria for mood disorders.[13,89] A similar incidence of depression can be seen among opiate addicts. However, 20% of cocaine abusers experience cyclical mood disorders such as bipolar disorders (manic-depressive illness) and cyclothymic disorder; the incidence of these conditions in opiate addicts is only 1%. Such findings suggest that people who experience mood swings prefer stimulants over other illicit drugs. Another commonly seen condition among cocaine patients is residual attention-deficit disorder (hyperactivity).

Anxiety Disorders

In one national survey, 50% of callers reported experiencing cocaine-induced panic attacks. Treatment facilities specializing in panic and anxiety disorders also report that onset of panic attacks often begins with cocaine use.[90] Based on the observations of Uhde and associates, Post and colleagues have suggested that cocaine-induced panic attacks may develop in a manner similar to pharmacological kindling.[91] Specifically, cocaine-induced panic attacks may emerge and grow more common following long periods of repeated and intermittent cocaine use. Given enough repetitions of cocaine-induced panic attacks, a stage may develop whereby the panic attacks occur spontaneously—without the presence of cocaine. Interestingly, procaine— a compound that shares the local anesthetic properties of cocaine but not its stimulant effects—also activates the limbic system in a manner similar to cocaine.[92] Lidocaine, another local anesthetic without stimulant properties, has been associated with doom anxiety.[93] Therefore, a number of clinical manifestations of cocaine use may result from cocaine's local anesthetic properties and not its stimulant effect.

Personality Disorders

People with borderline personality disorder may use mood-altering drugs in a vain attempt at relief. They may use stimulants to induce feelings of pleasure or depressants to reduce internal distress. Because these people are already on edge, use of stimulants and depressants may trigger a flareup of anger or violence.

Perhaps more than any other personality disorder, people diagnosed as having antisocial disorder are prone to use mood-altering drugs. Alcohol is often the drug of choice in such individuals, but many also use cocaine or amphetamines or a combination of several drugs. People with this disorder are distressed, tense, unable to tolerate boredom, and agitated to the point of discomfort. Their use of drugs often removes any remaining inhibitions, increasing the risk of anger, violence, and actions that violate the rights or property of others. Because cocaine is by definition an illicit substance, use of the drug in itself constitutes a form of antisocial behavior.

Dissociative Disorders

Like a person with schizophrenia, a person experiencing cocaine delirium may lose contact with reality and become confused and disoriented. Auditory hallucinations and paranoia are traits commonly seen in both schizophrenia and cocaine abuse. The delirium of cocaine usually dissipates within a few days, although some symptoms of delirium may persist for up to a year.[94]

Eating Disorders

Many women with anorexia and bulimia take amphetamines to suppress the appetite. Some of these people progress to using cocaine or methamphetamine. One study of 386 consecutive patients admitted for inpatient substance abuse treatment found that 15% of 143 female patients had a lifetime diagnosis of anorexia or bulimia compared to only 1% of males.[95] In this study, women substance abusers with eating disorders were far more likely to abuse stimulants (82%) than opiates (5%). The preference for stimulants in this population suggests (1) a common psychopathology between stimulant abuse and eating disorders; (2) a preference for stimulants among eating disorder patients as a means of controlling appetite; or (3) a combination of the above factors. Chapter 9 discusses eating disorders and substance abuse in greater detail.

Medical Complications of Polydrug Abuse

The National Household Survey, conducted by NIDA, indicates that the 1-year prevalence of simultaneous cocaine and alcohol use is 4.7% in the general population.[96] Given that the 1-year prevalence of cocaine use is only 1.5% higher, one may conclude that the majority of cocaine users also use alcohol concurrently.

In 1991, researchers at the University of Miami School of Medicine found that a third substance called cocaethylene may result when cocaine and alcohol are mixed.[97] Cocaethylene increases both the euphoria and the craving associated with cocaine, while potentially increasing the risk of sudden death. In this study, medical examiners and researchers examined cocaine-related fatalities and found that cocaethylene occurred in 62% of the deaths where cocaine and alcohol were consumed. The cocaine-alcohol combination was found in over 52% of all cocaine-related fatalities. This study supports the findings of a Centers for Disease Control study which found that people with coronary disease who consume cocaine and alcohol have a 21.5 times greater risk of sudden death than those people who use only cocaine.

For example, cocaine when taken with marijuana increases heart rate and blood pressure to levels that surpass those reached by cocaine alone. Also, the combination of cocaine and alcohol increases the heart rate by a factor three to five times greater than either drug acting alone and greatly increases the chance of sudden death.

Routes of Administration

The clinical signs of cocaine abuse as well as a person's liability to cocaine addiction depend to a large degree on the route of administration. Other elements that determine addiction liability are the psychological and physical changes brought about by drug use, the degree of that change, the speed of onset of the change, the duration of change, and the postdrug effects.[98]

Cocaine tends to be less addictive if the dose is small, the peak plasma levels are low, the onset of activity is slow, the duration of action is long, and the unpleasant withdrawal effects are absent or very mild. Indeed, the addiction potential is lower if cocaine is taken by chewing coca leaves, through oral ingestion, or, to some extent, through intranasal use. Swallowing or snorting cocaine is an inefficient way of using the drug, since cocaine penetrates biological membranes poorly. Hepatic biotransformation prevents 70 to 80% of the oral or intranasal dose from reaching the circulatory system.[98]

After oral administration, cocaine concentrations in the blood rise slowly, peaking approximately 1 hour after ingestion. Behavioral effects of the drug tend to follow the same curve. In contrast, intranasal use produces a quicker onset of drug effects, shorter duration of action, and higher peak blood levels. Thus the addiction potential of intranasal cocaine abuse is higher than that of oral use largely because of the more rapid onset of pharmacological effects.

Intravenous cocaine use ranks higher on the addiction potential scale than intranasal use. Given unlimited access to the drug, IV cocaine abusers will escalate the dose until they deteriorate physically and mentally. The onset of the IV cocaine "rush" is within 30 to 45 seconds, and the drug's effects last for 10 to 20 minutes. Peak blood levels can be more than twice those that occur following intranasal ingestion. What's more, 100% of an IV dose is delivered to the circulatory system, compared to 20 to 30% of a snorted dose.[98] For many reasons—pain of injection, difficulty of finding and using needles and syringes, and risk of infectious disease—IV administration is less appealing to cocaine abusers than other methods.

Given the parameters that define addiction liability, cocaine in smokable form has the highest addictive potential. Cocaine can be smoked as coca paste, as freebase, or as crack, which is simply freebase prepared by a different method. The popularity of crack compared to freebase is largely a product of marketing techniques that make small amounts of high-quality cocaine available at low prices and without having to undertake a dangerous chemical process to convert cocaine to a smokable form.

In actuality, smoking is not an efficient system for delivering cocaine to the body. A significant portion of the drug dose is lost to pyrolysis. Nonetheless, the remaining dose produces potent effects. The resulting high is intense—some users describe it as "full body orgasm." The onset is extremely rapid; only 8 to 10 seconds elapse before the user experiences the high. The concentration of the drug in the brain also occurs more rapidly than following IV use, resulting in greater behavioral effects.

Also contributing to the addiction potential of crack

is the fact that the effects of the drug last only 5 to 10 minutes. After the high is over, the crack user feels anxious, depressed, and paranoid. Such a rapid shift between positive and negative effects of the drug make users crave another "hit" of the drug to restore the euphoria they felt just moments before. These cravings form a distinct part of the withdrawal syndrome associated with cocaine.

Withdrawal symptoms manifest as the inverse of the cocaine's effects. Such symptoms include decreased energy, limited interest in the environment, and limited ability to experience pleasure. These symptoms are mildest immediately following cessation of cocaine use but increase in intensity during the next 12 to 96 hours.[13]

For years people assumed cocaine was not addictive because it did not produce symptoms of withdrawal. We know now that extinguishing drug cravings is one of the most difficult aspects of treating the cocaine addict.

References

1. Jacobson SW, Jacobson JL, Sokol RJ, et al. Maternal recall of alcohol, cocaine, and marijuana use during pregnancy. *Neurotoxicol Teratol*. 1991;13:535–540.
2. Wallach MB, Gerson S. A neuropsychopharmacological comparison of d-amphetamine, L-dopa and cocaine. *Neuropharmacology*. 1971;10:743.
3. Dimijian GG. Contemporary drug abuse. In: Goth A, ed. *Medical Pharmacology, Principles and Concepts*. 7th ed. St. Louis: CV Mosby Co; 1974:313.
4. Sterk C. Cocaine and HIV seropositivity. *Lancet*. 1988;1:1052–1053.

5. Dackis CA, Gold MS. Biological aspects of cocaine addiction. In: Volkow ND, ed. *Cocaine in the Brain*. Houston: Rutgers University Press; 1988.

6. Mule SJ. The pharmacodynamics of cocaine abuse. *Psychiatric Ann*. 1984;14(10):724–727.

7. Gold MS, Verebey K. The psychopharmacology of cocaine. *Psychiatric Ann*. 1984;14(10):714–723.

8. Gawin FH, Ellinwood EH Jr. Cocaine and other stimulants. *N Engl J Med*. 1988;318(18):1173–1182.

9. Weinstein SP, Gottheil E, Smith RH, Migrala KA. Cocaine users seen in medical practice. *Am J Drug Alcohol Abuse*. 1986;12:341–354.

10. Jeri FR, Sanchez CC, Del Pozo T, Fernandez M, Carbajal C. Further experience with the syndromes produced by coca paste smoking. In: Jeri FR, ed. *Cocaine 1980*. Lima, Peru: Pacific Press; 1980.

11. Jaffee JH. Drug addiction and drug abuse. In: Goodman AG, Gilman LS, eds. *The Pharmacological Basis of Therapeutics*. 7th ed. New York: Macmillan; 1985:532–581.

12. Anthony JC, Tien AY, Petronis KR. Epidemiologic evidence on cocaine use and panic attacks. *Am J Epidemiol*. 1989; 129(3):543–549.

13. Gawin FH, Kleber HD. Abstinence symptomatology and psychiatric diagnosis in cocaine abusers: clinical observations. *Arch Gen Psychiatry*. 1986;43:107–113.

14. Marzuk PM, Tardiff K, Leon AC, Stajic M, Morgan EB, Mann JJ. Prevalence of recent cocaine use among motor vehicle fatalities in New York City. *JAMA*. 1990;263(2):250–256.

15. Novick DM. The medically ill substance abuser. In: Lowinson JH, et al. eds. *Substance Abuse: A Comprehensive Textbook*. Baltimore, Md: Williams & Wilkins; 1992:chap 50.

16. Benchimol A, Bartall H, Desser KB. Accelerated ventricular rhythm and cocaine abuse. *Ann Intern Med*. 1978;88:519–520.

17. Karch SB, Billingham ME. The pathology and etiology of cocaine-induced heart disease. *Arch Pathol Lab Med*. 1988;112(3):225–230.

18. Crumb WJ Jr, Clarkson CW. Characterization of cocaine-induced block of cardiac sodium channels. *Biophys J*. 1990: 57(3):589–599.

19. Jones LF, Tackett RL. Central mechanisms of action involved in cocaine-induced tachycardia. *Life Sci.* 1990;46(10):723–728.

20. Perez-Meyes M, DiGuiseppi S, Ondrusek G, Jeffcoat AR, Cook CE. Free-base cocaine smoking. *Clin Pharmacol Ther.* 1982;32:459–465.

21. Foltin RW, Fischman MW, Pedroso JJ, Pearlson GD. Repeated intranasal cocaine administration: lack of tolerance to pressor effects. *Drug Alcohol Depend.* 1988;22:169–177.

22. Lichtenfeld PJ, Rubin DB, Feldman RS. Subarachnoid hemorrhage precipitated by cocaine snorting. *Arch Neurol.* 1984;41:223–224.

23. Fredericks RK, Lefkowitz DS, Challa VR, Troost BT. Cerebral vasculitis associated with cocaine abuse. *Stroke.* November 1991;22(11):1437–1439.

24. Smith HWB, Lieberman HA, Brody SL, Battey LL, Donohue BC, Morris DC. Acute myocardial infarction temporally related to cocaine use. *Ann Intern Med.* 1987;107:13–18.

25. Vitullo JC, Karam R, Mekhail N, Wicker P, Engelmann A, Khairallah PA. Cocaine-induced small vessel spasm in isolated rat hearts. *Am J Pathol.* 1989;135(1):85–91.

26. Isner HM, Estes NAM III, Thompson PD, et al. Acute cardiac events temporally related to cocaine abuse. *N Engl J Med.* 1986;315:1438–1443.

27. Amin M, Gabelman G. Cocaine and chest pain. *Ann Intern Med.* 1992;116(1):91. Letter.

28. Wilkerson RD. Cardiovascular toxicity of cocaine. In: Clouet D, Asghar K, Brown R, eds. *Natl Inst Drug Abuse Res Monogr Ser.* 1988;88:304–324.

29. Nadamanee K, Gorelick DA, Josephson MA, et al. Myocardial ischemia during cocaine withdrawal. *Ann Intern Med.* 1989;111(11):876–880.

30. Schachne JS, Roberts BH, Thompson PD. Coronary-artery spasm and myocardial infarction associated with cocaine use. *N Engl J Med.* 1984;310:1665–1666.

31. Dressler FA, Malekzadeh S, Roberts WC, et al. Quantitative analysis of amounts of coronary arterial narrowing in cocaine addicts. *JAMA.* 1990;263(23):3197.

32. Togna G, Tempesta E, Togna AR, Doci N, Cebo B, Caprino I. Platelet responsiveness and biosynthesis of thromboxane pro-

stacyclin in response in in vitro cocaine treatment. *Haemostasis.* 1985;15:100–107.

33. Peng SK, French WJ, Pelikan PCD. Direct cocaine cardiotoxicity demonstrated by endomyocardial biopsy. *Arch Pathol Lab Med.* 1989;113(8):842–845.

34. Wiener MD, Putnam CE. Pain in the chest in a user of cocaine. *JAMA.* 1987;258(15):2087–2088.

35. Itkonen J, Schnoll A, Glassroth J. Pulmonary dysfunction in "freebase" cocaine users. *Arch Intern Med.* 1984;144:2195–2197.

36. Hoffman CK, Goodman PC. Pulmonary edema in cocaine smokers. *Radiology.* 1989;172(2):462–465.

37. Cregler LL, Mark H. Medical complications of cocaine abuse. *N Engl J Med.* 1986;315:1495–1500.

38. Murray RJ, Albin RJ, Mergner W, et al. Diffuse alveolar hemorrhage temporally related to cocaine smoking. *Chest.* 1988;427–429

39. Rebhum J. Association of asthma and freebase smoking. *Ann Allergy.* 1988;60(4):339–342.

40. Jonsson S, O'Meara M, Young JB. Acute cocaine poisoning: importance of treating seizures and acidosis. *Am J Med.* 1983; 75:1061–1064.

41. Barden JC. Crack smoking seen as a peril to the lungs. *New York Times.* December 24, 1989:19.

42. Byck R. *Cocaine Papers: Sigmund Freud.* New York: Stonehill Publishing Co; 1974.

43. Merriam AE, Medalia A, Levine B. Partial complex status epilepticus associated with cocaine abuse. *Biol Psychiatry.* 1988;23:515–518.

44. Post RM, Kopanda RT, Black KE. Progressive effects of cocaine on behavior and central amine metabolism in the rhesus monkey: relationship to kindling and psychosis. *Biol Psychiatry.* 1976;11:403–419.

45. Estroff TW, Gold MS. Chronic medical complications of drug abuse. *Psychiatric Med.* 1987;3(3):267–286.

46. Ashley R. *Cocaine: Its History, Uses and Effects.* New York: St. Martin's Press; 1975:240.

47. Siegel RK. Cocaine smoking. *J Pyschoactive Drugs.* 1982;14:277–359.

48. Smith DE, Wesson DR, Apter-Marsh M. Cocaine- and alcohol-

induced sexual dysfunction in patients with addictive diseases. *J Psychoactive Drugs*. 1984;16:359–361.

49. Chasnoff IJ, Burns WJ, Schnoll SH, Burns KA. Cocaine use in pregnancy. *N Engl J Med*. 1985;313:666–669.
50. Centers for Disease Control. HIV/AIDS surveillance: AIDS cases reported through September 1989. Washington, DC: U.S. Department of Health and Human Services, Public Health Service; October 1989.
51. Mendelson J, Teoh S, Lange U, Mello N, Weiss R, Skupny A. Hyperprolactinemia during cocaine withdrawal. In: Harris LS, ed. *Natl Inst Drug Abuse Res Monogr Sr*. 1988;81:67–73.
52. Jonas JM, Gold MS. Cocaine abuse and eating disorders. *Lancet*. 1986;1:390–391.
53. Ritchie JM, Greene NM. Local anesthetics. In: Gilman AG, Goodman LS, Rall TW, et al., eds. *The Pharmacological Basis of Therapeutics*. 7th ed. New York: Macmillan; 1985:309–310.
54. Roberts DCS, Quattrocchi E, Howland MA. Severe hyperthermia secondary to intravenous drug abuse. *Am J Emerg Med*. 1984;2:373.
55. Loghmanee F, Tobak M. Fatal malignant hyperthermia associated with recreational cocaine and ethanol abuse. *Am J Forensic Med Pathol*. 1986;7(3):246–248.
56. Goldfrank LR, et al., eds. *Toxicologic Emergencies*. 3rd ed. Norwalk, Conn: Appleton-Century-Crofts; 1986:477–486.
57. Gold MS. Medical implications of cocaine intoxication. *Alcoholism and Addiction*. October 1989:16.
58. Merigian KS, Roberts JR. Cocaine intoxication: hyperpyrexia, rhabdomyolysis, and acute renal failure. *J Toxicol Clin Toxicol*. 1987;25:135–148.
59. Krohn KD, Slowman-Kovacs S, Leapman SB. Cocaine and rhabdomyolysis. *Ann Intern Med*. 1988;208:639–640.
60. Roth D, Alarcon FJ, Fernandez JA, Preston RA, Bourgoignie JJ. Acute rhabdomyolysis associated with cocaine intoxication. *N Engl J Med*. 1988;319(11):673–677.
61. Nolte KB. Rhabdomyolysis associated with cocaine abuse. *Hum Pathol*. 1991;22:1141–1145.
62. Schweitzer VG. Osteolytic sinusitis and pneumomediastinum: deceptive otolaryngologic complications of cocaine abuse. *Laryngoscope*. 1986;96:206–210.

63. Vilensky W. Illicit and licit drugs causing perforation of the nasal septum. *J Forensic Sci.* 1982;27:958–962.
64. Van Dyke C, Jatlow P, Ungerer J, et al. Oral cocaine: plasma concentrations and central effects. *Science.* 1978;200:211–213.
65. Kreek MJ. Multiple drug abuse patterns and medical consequences. In: Meltzer HY, ed. *Psychopharmacology: The Third Generation of Progress.* New York: Raven Press; 1987:1600–1603.
66. Cregler LL, Mark H. Cardiovascular dangers of cocaine abuse. *Am J Cardiol.* 1986;57(1):1185–1186.
67. Kosten TR, Kleber HD. Sudden death in cocaine abusers: relation to neuroleptic malignant syndrome. *Lancet.* 1987;1(8543):1198–1199.
68. Kilaru P, Kim W, Sequeira W. Cocaine and scleroderma: is there an association? *J Rheumatol.* 1991;18:1753–1755.
69. Derlet RW, Albertson TE. Emergency department presentation of cocaine intoxication. *Ann Emerg Med.* 1989;18(2):115–119.
70. Chasnoff IJ, Griffith DR, Freier C, Murray J. Cocaine/polydrug use in pregnancy. *Pediatrics.* 1992;89(2):284–289.
71. George SK, Price J, Hauth J, Barnette DM, Preston P. Drug abuse screening of childbearing-age women in Alabama public health clinics. *Am J Obstet Gynecol.* 1991;165:924–927.
72. Woods JR Jr, Plessinger MA. Pregnancy increases cardiovascular toxicity to cocaine. *Am J Obstet Gynecol.* 1990;162(2):529–533.
73. Pritchard JA, MacDonald PC, Gant NF. *Williams Obstetrics.* Norwalk, Conn: Appleton-Century-Crofts; 1985:395–407.
74. Finnegan L. The dilemma of cocaine exposure in the perinatal period. *Natl Inst Drug Abuse Res Monogr Ser.* 1988;81:379.
75. Richards IS, Kulkarni AP, Remner WF. Cocaine-induced arrhythmia in human foetal myocardium in vitro: possible mechanism for foetal death in utero. *Pharmacol Toxicol.* 1990;66:150–154.
76. Tabor BL, Soffici AR, Smith-Wallace T, Yonekura ML. The effect of maternal cocaine use on the fetus: changes in antepartum fetal heart rate tracings. *Am J Obstet Gynecol.* 1991;165:1278–1281.
77. Hadeed AJ, Siegel SR. Maternal cocaine use during pregnancy: effect on the newborn infant. *Pediatrics.* 1989;84(2):205–210.
78. Critchley HOD, Woods SM, Barson AJ, et al. Fetal death in

utero and cocaine abuse. Case report. *Br J Obstet Gynecol.* 1988;95:195–196.

79. Bateman DA, Heagarty MC. Passive freebase cocaine ("crack") inhilation by infants and toddlers. *Am J Dis Child.* 1989; 134(1):25–27.

80. Dobersczak TM, Shanzer S, Senie RT, Kandall SR. Neonatal neurologic and electroencephalographic effects of intrauterine cocaine exposure. *J Pediatr.* 1988;113(2):354–358.

81. Zuckerman B, Frank DA, Hingson R, et al. Effects of maternal marijuana and cocaine use on fetal growth. *N Engl J Med.* 1989;320(12):762–768.

82. Newald J. Cocaine infants: a new arrival at hospital's step? *Hospitals.* 1986;60(7):96.

83. Astley SJ, Clarren SK, Little RE, Sampson PD, Daling JR. Analysis of facial shape in children gestationally exposed to marijuana, alcohol, and/or cocaine. *Pediatrics.* 1992;89:67–77.

84. Ward SLD, Schuetz S, Krishna V, et al. Abnormal sleeping ventilatory pattern in infants of substance-abusing mothers. *Am J Dis Child.* 1986;140:1015–1020.

85. Chasnoff IJ. Perinatal effects of cocaine. *Contemp OB/GYN.* May 1987:163–179.

86. Chasnoff IJ. Cocaine intoxication in an infant via maternal milk. *Pediatrics.* In press.

87. Infants, children test positive for cocaine after exposure to second-crack smoke. *JAMA Med News Perspect.* 1992;267(8):1044–1045.

88. Gold MS. *1988 Medical and Health Annual.* Chicago: Encyclopaedia Britannica, Inc; 1988:277–284.

89. Weiss RD, Mirin SM, Michael JL, Sollogub AC. Psychopathology in chronic cocaine abusers. *Am J Drug Alcohol Abuse.* 1986;12:17–29.

90. Gold MS. *The Good News About Panic, Anxiety, and Phobias.* New York: Villard Books; 1989.

91. Post RM, Weiss SB, Pert A. Sensitization and kindling effects of chronic cocaine administration. In: Lakowski JM, Galloway MP, Ehite FJ, eds. *Cocaine: Pharmacology, Physiology, and Clinical Strategies.* Boca Raton, Fla: CRC Press; 1992:chap 7.

92. Post R. Talk given at the ASAM's 23rd Annual Medical-Scientific Conference. Washington, DC; April 2–5, 1992.

93. Saravey SM, Marie J, Steinberg MD, Rabiner CJ. "Doom anxiety" and delirium in lidocaine toxicity. *Am J Psychiatry.* 1986;144:159.
94. Siegel RK. Cocaine smoking disorders: diagnosis and treatment. *Psychiatric Ann.* 1984;14(10):728–732.
95. Hudson JI, Weiss RD, Pope HG, McElroy SK, Mirin SM. Eating disorders in hospitalized substance abusers. *Am J Drug Alcohol Abuse.* 1992;18(1):75–85.
96. Katz JL, Terry P, Witkin JM. Comparative behavioral pharmacology and toxicology of cocaine and its ethanol-derived metabolite, cocaine ethyl-ester (cocaethylene). *Life Sci.* 1992;50:1351–1361.
97. Randall T. Cocaine, alcohol, mix in body to form even longer lasting, more lethal drug. *JAMA.* 1992;267(6):1043–1044.
98. Verebey K, Gold MS. From coca leaves to crack: the effects of dose and routes of administration in abuse liability. *Psychiatric Ann.* 1988;18(9):513–521.

5

Outpatient Treatment

The evaluation and initial treatment of cocaine-using patients is a complex, demanding, and sometimes confusing process. Thorough treatment requires the physician to integrate a range of medical, psychiatric, social, and drug-counseling services. Adding to the complexity is the need to address family issues and to anticipate the risk of relapse. Treatment can be expensive, but a recent study found that for every treatment dollar spent, $11.54 was saved in social costs (the costs to society from arrests, prosecution, theft, medical care, impaired job performance, and so on).[1] Although currently the success rate of treatment for drug addiction is less than would be desired, new treatment strategies, including some pharmacological interventions, offer hope for improving the outcome.

Specific treatment programs designed for cocaine users are a relatively new development. In fact, a 1979 chapter on cocaine by Grinspoon and Bakalar (in the

Handbook of Drug Abuse, published by the National Institute on Drug Abuse) does not even mention the subject of cocaine abuse treatment.[2] The cocaine epidemic
of the 1980s shattered this naive and inaccurate view of
cocaine and necessitated cocaine treatment programs.

By 1991, the National Household Survey estimated
that 23.7 million Americans had used cocaine at least
once in their lifetime and that 1.9 million were current
users (at least once in the last 30 days).[3] Approximately
22 million, or 92% of the people who have used cocaine, are not currently using it. Of these 22 million
people, only a small fraction have ever entered into a
treatment program. Although it is impossible to determine exactly why over 20 million people chose not to
continue their cocaine use, public attitudes about the
dangers of cocaine surely have played a significant role
in limiting the number of current users. Physicians
who have recognized the importance of detecting substance abuse and who have attempted to educate their
patients and the public about the dangers of drug
abuse are to be commended. However, numerous problems still exist in the manner in which the medical
profession treats substance abuse.[4]

Clearly, the physician's role in identifying drug
users and encouraging drug treatment should not be
underestimated. A recent study of alcoholic workers
in an employee assistance program after their drug
use had been identified on the job attempted to discern
the importance of a physician's warning in treatment
success.[5] This study found that 74% of the alcoholic
workers had seen a physician during the year prior to
their intake into the treatment program. Of these patients, however, only 22% could remember any physi-

cian warning—even though their alcohol consumption was significant enough to be identified by company and union supervisors. After 2 years, the ability to remember the physician's warning was associated with a significantly better prognosis and treatment outcome. The results of this study confirm other reports of physician failure to adequately detect substance abuse and direct their patients to the proper treatment program.

Cocaine Treatment Programs

In recent years, many cocaine treatment programs have adopted the chemical dependency model, which regards drug dependence as a disease unto itself and not merely as a secondary problem arising from some other underlying psychiatric condition. Such programs take a multidisciplinary approach to drug treatment and provide a range of behavioral, cognitive, educational, and self-control techniques aimed at reduction of drug cravings and the potential for relapse. It is significant that the majority of these programs also require patients to abstain from all drugs and to participate actively in Twelve Step programs such as Alcoholics Anonymous (AA) or Cocaine Anonymous (CA). The advantage of these Twelve Step programs is that patients learn to consider themselves as being continually at risk and in a recovering—rather than a recovered—state. They also learn to see themselves as chemically dependent, not mentally ill. Such a fundamental shift in perspective improves the chances that the patient will live a drug-free life. One study found a treatment success rate of 90% one year after leaving treatment programs for patients who combined AA participation with an aftercare program.[6] By comparison, treatment success rates of approximately 70% were achieved by patients who attended either AA or aftercare programs, but not both.

Ideally, all addicts, having recognized how drugs have ruined their lives, would voluntarily enter a treatment program. Unfortunately, this ideal notion is at odds with the clandestine nature of addiction. Many addicts who "volunteer" to enter a treatment program often do so in an attempt to control, and not abolish, their drug use. These patients may leave a treatment program if their drug use is significantly threatened.

Other addicts voluntarily enter treatment after "bottoming out." Their drug use has devastated their lives, destroyed their homes, and wrecked their jobs—in short, they have reached bottom. Although treatment for these individuals can succeed, it is extremely difficult. These "bottomed-out" addicts usually have no support, either financial, familial, social, or work-related, to help them through the difficult task of recovery.

Interestingly, patients who are forced to enter treatment programs, either through the criminal system, family intervention, or workplace drug screens, may fare better than patients who voluntarily enter treatment. For example, a study of drug-dependent criminal offenders found that the criminals who were forced to undergo treatment had lower rates of crime and unemployment 7 years after their release than did the criminals who were not forced to receive drug treatment. Other studies have found that patients entering treatment under legal pressure did at least as well, and in some cases better, than voluntary patients. Patients forced to enter treatment often do better because they have a reason—to keep their job and/or their family or even to stay out of prison. Often, this reason keeps patients in treatment longer.[7]

When patients enter the health care system, on either a voluntary or forced basis, the first step they encounter is diagnosis. Diagnosis is essential not only to detect any underlying psychological or physical conditions (see preceding chapters) but also to gauge the extent of a person's drug use. Unfortunately, many health care providers rely on patient self-reports rather than using drug screens as a means of confirming a history of drug use or detecting recent use in patients who deny using drugs. Self-reported drug use is notoriously unreliable, as patients frequently conceal or underestimate their drug consumption. In addition to drug screens, physicians should take a detailed patient and family history while observing the patient carefully for any of the signs of cocaine dependence (see Table 5.1).

In addition, the patient should undergo a thorough physical and laboratory examination. HIV and hepatitis testing, chest X-rays, electrocardiograms, and other indicated procedures may supply life-saving information and/or may help to reassure patients about their state of health. Any severe conditions or impending medical emergencies may result in the patient being transferred to a medical hospital.

The quantity and frequency of cocaine consumed, the route of administration (intravenous, smoking, or sniffing), the existence and extent of other drug or alcohol abuse, past attempts at treatment, and the mental and physical health of the patient all play important roles in determining whether the patient would benefit

TABLE 5.1. Diagnostic Criteria for Cocaine Dependency[11]

Loss of control
Inability to stop using or to refuse cocaine
Failure to self-limit use
Predictable or regular use
Binges for 24 hours or longer
Urges and cravings for cocaine
Exaggerated involvement
Self-proclaimed need for cocaine
Fear of distress without cocaine
Feelings of dependency on cocaine
Feelings of guilt about using cocaine and fear of being discovered
Preference for cocaine over family, friends, and recreational activities
Continued use despite adverse effects
Medical problems (e.g., fatigue, insomnia, headaches, nasal problems, bronchitis)
Psychological problems (e.g., irritability, depression, loss of sex drive, lack of motivation, memory impairment)
Social/interpersonal problems (e.g., loss of friends or spouse, job difficulties, social withdrawal, involvement in traffic accidents, excuse-making behavior)

best by outpatient or inpatient treatment or whether another form of treatment is indicated.

Most cocaine treatment programs in this country fall into one of five categories:

- *Outpatient clinics* provide counseling and support for people trying to overcome their drug use while they continue to live and function within the community.
- *Self-help groups,* such as Cocaine Anonymous, may be the first form of treatment a cocaine addict will encounter. In addition, many outpa-

tient and inpatient programs stress participation in self-help groups as an essential component of a successful recovery.

- *Residential therapeutic communities* are highly structured programs lasting up to 18 months in which addicts live together while working to change the habits and attitudes that contribute to their drug problems. Phoenix House and Daytop Village are well-known examples of this type of treatment.
- *Detoxification programs* are those in which patients stay in a care facility for a few days with the specific goal of detoxification.
- *Chemical dependency programs* are usually private inpatient units in hospitals or other facilities where treatment usually lasts up to 4 weeks. These programs offer patients a range of other supportive therapies in addition to detoxification.

If circumstances permit, outpatient treatment is the preferred treatment method for several reasons. The majority of cocaine abusers can be treated as outpatients, since use of the drug can usually be stopped abruptly without medical risk or significant discomfort. The goal of treatment is to return the patient to a normal life; by definition there can be no "normal" life inside the hospital. Many patients are more willing to accept help on an outpatient basis, since it carries less of a social stigma and is less disruptive to daily life. Given the rising demand for treatment, there may be more outpatient treatment slots available.

The standards for a good outpatient treatment program are shown in Table 5.2. Most important, this program should make sure that the program advocates *complete abstinence from all drugs.* The treatment program must also advocate *regular drug testing.* Ideally, urine samples should be collected two or three times a week to ensure patient compliance with the treatment regimen. Far from being invasive, such testing actually works to build trust between the patient and the caregiver, since drug testing should remove the caregiver's doubts about the patient's abstinence while giving the patient an objective means to verify his or her compliance with the treatment program. Therefore, drug testing helps to eliminate the denial and self-deceit that so often sabotage treatment.[8]

In conjunction with drug testing, the program must clearly spell out the *consequences for failure.* Among the possibilities are temporary suspension from the program; more frequent therapy sessions; more intensive education; or admission (in some cases, readmission) to a hospital.

Outpatient therapy has to be chosen carefully to

TABLE 5.2. Characteristics of Model Outpatient Programs[12]

Advocate total abstinence from all mood-altering drugs
Present accurate and current information about the health hazards of drug use
Encourage the patient to change but do not resort to lectures or harangues
Address the patient's age, interests, and special needs
Involve parents, spouses, or other important people
Emphasize the present impact of drug use and hold patients accountable for their actions
Use urine testing to assure and monitor compliance

---

address an individual person's problems. Patients may need some combination of vocation rehabilitation, family therapy, or couples therapy. The people who are important in a patient's life need to learn what roles they should play in recovery. They may need to be taught, for example, to withhold money from the patient or to avoid acting as enablers for the patient's destructive behavior. The younger the patient, the more important it is that the entire family become involved in treatment.

As for structure, the best programs recognize the different (and, to a degree, overlapping) phases of addiction and recovery and will offer support at each of these steps along the road to recovery.

The first phase is abstinence. For the first 30 to 60 days of treatment, work focuses on making patients drug free. Although this goal is both realistic and achievable, abstinence in an outpatient setting may provoke withdrawal symptoms or intense cravings for cocaine. These cravings are often the result of exposure to conditioned cues ("people, places, or things") that ignite memories of cocaine euphoria. To help ensure compliance, the patient should see the therapist frequently during this phase to get counseling, support, and education.

Addicts need to learn that drug use is largely a conditioned response and that exposure to objects (such as talcum powder), a drug-using friend, an environment associated with past drug use, or even emotional states may trigger cravings. A good treatment program recognizes the power of these stimuli, warns patients about them, and teaches techniques for controlling them.

At some point, gradually and under supervision, patients must return to settings where triggers exist, and they must do so without succumbing to drug urges. Long-term support, Twelve-Step participation, and/or peer-group therapy can be beneficial in helping patients make this transition.

The emphasis during this second phase is now on anticipating and preventing relapse. To reach this goal and make the necessary changes in life-style, patients need education and support. The danger of relapse has to be acknowledged and confronted. Denying the threat of relapse means the program has no policy for dealing with it when it erupts.

Some of the techniques for preventing relapse include predicting which situations are more likely to trigger cravings; rehearsing strategies for avoiding those situations or for responding to them without resorting to drugs; altering life-style—changing jobs, for example, if necessary; developing drug-free support networks; reinforcing the negative aspects and painful memories of drug use; and working to reduce or cope with stress.[9]

The final phase arrives usually a year or so after treatment begins and continues indefinitely afterward. By this point, patients have learned which strategies work for them and which don't. Often they then graduate to self-help programs or therapy groups that have a different focus. Early in abstinence, the emphasis was on the day-to-day struggle against drugs; now it's on the long-term aspects of a drug-free life. One goal, for example, is to combat overconfidence, a feeling that often emerges after a patient has managed to avoid drugs for a few months. Also, people may need help coping with the psychological problems that may emerge once their drug use has ceased.

Group Therapy

A good outpatient treatment program is one that first works to help the patient become abstinent and drug free. At some point in that process, patients will be ready to benefit from self-help groups like AA or CA and a structured, medically supervised group therapy. In group sessions, addicts get the chance to express their feelings about their drug urges and the way drugs have affected their thinking. They can trade ideas on ways to avoid relapse.[10] In group therapy, patients learn that others share their problems and that they are not alone in their struggle. In the process they realize that it's possible to develop and adopt an entirely new belief system, one that isn't founded on the use of drugs.

To be most effective, group therapy sessions should adhere to the following "group rules." Patients should understand from the very beginning that violation of these rules may lead to immediate termination from the group and even from the treatment program itself.

1. You are expected to come to group sessions completely "straight," not under the influence of any mood-altering chemicals whatsoever.
2. You are expected to abstain from the use of alcohol and all other mood-altering chemicals during your participation in the group. In the event of relapse you must notify your counselor before attending the next group session,

and you must bring up the relapse episode for discussion at the beginning of the next group session. "Slips" will be viewed as potential learning experiences, but you will not be able to continue in the group if you show a regular pattern of slips, since this is destructive for you and for your fellow group members. If you are removed from the group due to slips, you will be given the option, where appropriate, of receiving three-times-a-week individual counseling to help you reestablish at least 2 consecutive weeks of uninterrupted abstinence as a prerequisite to applying for reentry into the group.

3. You agree to attend all scheduled sessions and to arrive on time without fail. This may require you to rearrange other obligations and perhaps even postpone vacations and out-of-town trips while participating in the group.

4. You agree to preserve the anonymity and confidentiality of all group members. You must not divulge the identity of any group member nor the content of any group discussions to persons outside the group.

5. You agree to remain in the group until you have completed the program. If you have an impulse or desire to leave the group prematurely, you will raise this issue for discussion in the group before acting on these feelings.

6. You agree to refrain throughout your participation in the program from becoming involved romantically, sexually, or financially with other group members.

7. You agree to accept immediate termination from

the program if you offer drugs or alcohol to any member of the group or use these substances together with another group member.

8. You agree to have your telephone number(s) added to the contact list distributed to all group members.

9. You agree to give a supervised urine sample at least twice a week and whenever the group leader may request it.

10. You agree to raise for discussion in the group any issue that threatens your own or another member's recovery. You will not keep secrets regarding another member's drug use or other destructive behavior.

The Role of Twelve-Step (Self-Help) Groups

Most recovering addicts find that Twelve-Step groups are an essential part of their abstinence. The phrase "Twelve-Step" refers to the fact that these groups follow in the tradition of Alcoholics Anonymous. Each Twelve-Step group is run completely by volunteers who are themselves recovering substance abusers. Members share their stories and explain their ways of surviving in the real world. Hearing such stories helps addicts to open up and share some of their own experiences. For an addict overwhelmed with shame, seeing so many other people with similar problems can be a tremendous relief and extremely therapeutic. Twelve-Step participation motivates people to stay drug free, while providing support if they slip.

Members of Twelve-Step groups admit, to themselves and others, that they cannot drink or use drugs.

In doing so they give up their illusion that they have control over their substance abuse. They replace that illusion with the reality—reinforced just by taking part in group sessions—that they are working to achieve self-mastery over their behavior.

In the past, there has been an unfortunate division between the medical and self-help communities. An underlying mistrust between psychiatry and self-help groups has developed largely because psychiatry has been hesitant to accept addictionology as a unique discipline, and self-help groups have resisted promoting the use of psychopharmacological agents.[8] In addition, there are important misconceptions that the psychiatrist is only useful for psychiatric conditions apart from addiction, despite "psychoactive substance use disorders" having full status in DSM-III-R. The psychiatrist is typically not employed in the primary treatment of addictive disorders but rather is an adjunct to assess "other psychiatric illness" in the addiction treatment populations. In many cases, the psychiatrist is called to evaluate or defend the need for medications. Moreover, there is the notion that the psychiatrist can play no role in the long-term recovery from addiction despite reports that recovering addicts use psychiatric and other services and view them as helpful. Table 5.3 summarizes the traditional approaches taken by self-help groups and psychiatry, as well as providing some common ground for compromise.

Residential Treatment

Residential treatment programs are akin to a combination of outpatient and inpatient programs. They

TABLE 5.3. Self-Help vs. Psychiatric Approaches[13]

Topic	Self-help view	Psychiatric view	Compromise
Drug-use cause	Drugs are used because individual is an addict	Complex dynamics influence behavior	First, stop drug use. Then confront emotional and psychological problems
Recovery	Follow the program	Extensive therapeutic work	Combine self-help participation with any necessary psychiatric care
AA/CA/NA, etc.	Life-saving gifts	Rigid, potentially harmful neglect of psychiatric issues	Appreciate the benefits of self-help groups while realizing their limitations
Controlled drinking	Impossible	May be possible	Impossible
Medication	Dangerous	Mends biological problems	Helpful during detox and for dual diagnosis when appropriately used
Psychopathology	Psychological problems result from drug use. Stop the drug use and problems stop	Specific conflicts may predate and cause drug use	Most often psychological problems are caused by drug use. However, dual diagnosis is a possibility
Treatment	Work the program	Medical and psychological	Combine medical, psychiatric, and self-help groups for best treatment outcomes
Treatment basis	Shared experience with others	Research combined with clinical observations	Integration of both approaches

129

are similar to inpatient programs in the sense that addicts agree to live with others in a therapeutic community for extended lengths of time—up to 2 years. But not all residential treatment programs are run by doctors, and they are thus not necessarily medical programs. They focus instead on helping patients learn, day by day, how to take responsibility for one's own life and for the lives of others within that community. In that sense, they are outpatient programs—therapy groups that live together 24 hours a day, using behavioral and cognitive methods to change their actions and attitudes.

Two of the best-known residential programs are Phoenix House and Daytop Village. Typically, a residential program may last 18 months, with residents beginning the program by working at menial tasks—sweeping, washing floors, cleaning bathrooms. Eventually they earn the right to take on more responsibility. At the same time they undergo intensive counseling to help them resist drugs. If they break any of the strict rules, they lose privileges, such as weekend leaves, and may be demoted from the favored jobs they had worked so hard to earn.

Residents participate in group discussion, job training seminars, and classes to prepare them for the graduate equivalency diplomas. Group sessions are the cornerstone of the program. During some sessions they may write and perform inspirational songs or skits. On weekends, things relax somewhat; there may be videos to watch or supervised trips off the premises.

These residential programs can bring about a deep and profound change in some members. They can be very effective and meaningful.

Follow-Up Care and Family Involvement

The last ingredient in the recipe for treatment is *follow-up care* through counseling and continuing access to therapy. It takes incredible stamina and willpower for recovering addicts to remain drug free; most find it impossible to avoid relapse entirely. Without ongoing support through follow-up care, they may not stand a chance. Treating the entire family should be an essential aspect of all follow-up programs.

Addiction is an illness that affects the entire family. Several years ago, this statement would have been ignored or scoffed at by the majority of treatment providers. Today, this concept has become an integral part of virtually every treatment program. In fact, this concept has become so ingrained in our society that many of the "buzz words" associated with it, such as codependency and enabling, have become a part of our everyday vocabulary. Often, however, familiarity with words obscures their true meaning.

Quite simply, a *codependent* is anyone directly involved with an addict's life—parents, spouse, children, even close friends. They are called codependents because their behavior and attitudes affect the patient, and the patient in turn affects them. Addicts are defined as dependents because of their reliance on a drug.

Though they may be completely unaware of it, codependents define their roles in life by their relationship to their loved one's addiction. The wife who works two jobs while her addicted husband remains unemployed and the older daughter who takes care of the younger children because the parents are too drunk are both examples of codependents. By their actions, these codependents may be *enabling* the addict's drug use to continue. Often codependents see themselves as "saviors" who have failed to save the addict from addiction. "If only I were a better spouse," their logic goes, "then my husband wouldn't have to use drugs."

When the addict tries to get help, the family may feel threatened. The life they've struggled to achieve, a life that is centered on the identified patient's addiction, is about to be lost. Thus, the codependents often interfere with the process of treatment—openly, through sabotage and denial, or covertly, by resisting their own need to change. Successful treatment programs must deal with these potential traps by educating and treating all family members about the dangers of codependency. Support groups such as *Alateen* and *Alanon* are excellent means of helping family members cope with the problems of addiction.

Left untreated, children in these families often grow up to have poor self-images and low self-esteem, and they may find it impossible to develop satisfactory relationships with others. They grow to mistrust all people but ironically feel more comfortable with intolerable behavior. This behavior is so common that the early 1980s saw the phenomenal growth of the grassroots movement *Adult Children of Alcoholics* (ACOAs).

Even if ACOAs themselves do not turn into alcoholics, they often suffer psychological problems. Through their constant search for approval from others, and by always placing other people's needs ahead of their own, ACOAs get used to living with dysfunctional people. Often one result is that they form similar abusive and codependent relationships.

ACOAs may find themselves unable to confront

their spouse's or child's drinking or drug problem directly. Instead, they do what they have always done: They try to control the other person's problems indirectly. They continue to lie, cover up, and clean up after the alcoholic, thinking that they do so out of love. Sometimes they harbor secret fantasies that through their loving patience, through their constant devotion, they will somehow cure their loved ones of their disease.

Without realizing it, though, they begin to define their whole identity in terms of their loved one's substance abuse problem. The dutiful wife or husband sees the spouse's problem as his or her cross to bear in life. The widespread attention given to the problems of ACOAs in the 1980s has helped millions of people to recognize their dysfunctional behavior and seek help either through self-help groups or with professional treatment.

References

1. Tabbush V. The effectiveness and efficiency of publicly funded drug abuse treatment and prevention programs in California: a benefit-cost analysis. UCLA Graduate School of Management, March 1986. As reported in "Treatment Works"; published by National Association of State Alcohol and Drug Abuse Directors; March 1990.
2. Grinspoon L, Bakalar JB. Cocaine. In: DuPont RL, Godstein A, O'Donnell J, eds. *Handbook of Drug Abuse*. Rockville Md: National Institute on Drug Abuse; 1979.
3. The 1991 National Household Survey. Rockville, Md: National Institute on Drug Abuse.
4. Bowe OP, Sammons JH. The alcohol-abusing patient: a challenge to the profession. *JAMA*. 1988;260:2267–2270.
5. Walsh D, Chapman Hingson RW, Merrigan DM, et al. The

impact of a physician's warning on recovery after alcoholism treatment. *JAMA* 1992;267(5):663–668.

6. Hoffman NG. Treatment outcomes from abstinence-based programs. Presented at the 36th International Institute on the Prevention and Treatment of Alcoholism; Stockholm, Sweden; June 1991.

7. Leukefeld CG. Opportunities for enhancing drug abuse treatment with criminal justice authority. National Institute on Drug Abuse Research Monograph #106: Improving Drug Abuse Treatment; 1991:328–337.

8. Gold MS. *The Good News About Drugs and Alcohol*. New York: Villard Books; 1991.

9. Gawin FH, Ellinwood EH Jr. Cocaine and other stimulants. *N Eng J Med*. 1988;318(18):1173–1182.

10. Gold MS. The cocaine epidemic: what are the problems, insights, and treatments? *Pharmacy Times*. March 1987:36–42.

11. Washton AM, et al. Opiate and cocaine dependencies: techniques to help counter the rising tide. *Postgrad Med*. 1985;77(5):293–300.

12. Adapted from Gold MS, et al. New treatments for opiate and cocaine users. *Psychiatric Ann*. 1986;16(4):208.

13. Nace EP. Alcoholics Anonymous. In Lowinson JH, Ruiz P, Millman RB, eds. *Substance Abuse: A Comprehensive Textbook*. 2nd ed. Baltimore, Md: Williams & Wilkins; 1992.

6

Inpatient Treatment and Relapse Prevention

Forty years ago there was only one drug addiction treatment center in the United States. By the late 1980s, there were approximately 9000 treatment programs serving nearly 600,000 addicts at any given time.[1] The recent decrease in overall drug use, coupled with our recent economic troubles, has significantly slowed the growth of treatment programs—nevertheless, specialized inpatient or outpatient treatment programs are still widely available.

The Benefits of Inpatient Care

When outpatient care is not possible, or has failed in the past, hospitalization can benefit the recovering patient, especially when combined with long-term par-

135

ticipation in self-help groups (such as AA). For example, a recent study found that inpatient treatment followed by mandatory AA attendance was twice as successful in achieving a 2-year abstinence when compared to AA alone or when patients chose their own recovery program[2] (see Figure 6.1).

Hospitalization helps because patients confined to a locked ward under continual care are denied access to drugs and their past drug-using environment. They can also take advantage of the many types of therapy (individual, group, creative, and so on) the hospital offers. Being in a therapeutic environment geared to helping them overcome their addiction shows patients that it is possible to become drug free and stay that way.

Another benefit is that doctors experienced in diagnosing and treating substance abuse can do full medical and psychiatric evaluations. Such observations

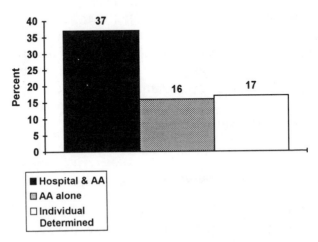

FIGURE 6.1. Abstinence rates after 2 years.

reveal whether the patient has any coexisting problems—medical problems or clinical depression, for example—that need additional treatment. Many of these problems emerge, and can be properly evaluated, only after detoxification and during observation over a period of several drug-free days.

Patient evaluation is an ongoing process that can be difficult for the physician who lacks experience in dealing with substance abuse patients. These physicians, expecting the physician-patient relationship to be a collaborative experience where the doctor listens to the patient and consults physical and laboratory evaluations while arriving at a differential diagnosis and treatment plan, may be unprepared for the deception and denial associated with substance abuse. Even families may misrepresent the patient's drug use (for example, a family member may claim that the patient "is doing much better since we first brought him in. He really doesn't need to be hospitalized"). In reality, the family member may be denying the real extent of the drug use and feeling guilty over the patient's hospitalization. Experienced clinicians can often help both the patient and the family to accurately assess the extent of the drug use.

Hospitalization may not be necessary for many patients. Patients who are highly motivated to get better, and who have a satisfying job and strong support among family, friends, or other social networks, may best benefit from outpatient programs. Similarly, outpatient treatment may be the preferred mode if the patient does not require detoxification or is in no immediate medical or psychiatric danger.

However, hospitalization can be called for in severe cases. Washton[3] lists the criteria for inpatient treatment as including:

- Chronic freebase or intravenous use.
- Concurrent dependency on other addictive drugs or alcohol.
- Serious medical or psychiatric problems.
- Severe impairment of psychological functioning.
- Insufficient motivation for outpatient treatment.
- Lack of family and social supports.
- Failure in outpatient treatment.

Since one great benefit of inpatient care is a thorough medical evaluation for comorbid and other disorders, as soon as possible after admission the patient should be seen by both an internist and a psychiatrist. This initial evaluation should be directed toward the stabilization of any existing medical problems and the detection of any other psychiatric condition. Table 6.1 lists the type of information that should be gleaned initially.

TABLE 6.1. Initial Screening Areas

1. What is the current cocaine abuse pattern?
2. What is the history of all drug abuse/use?
3. What is the current concomitant drug use?
4. Does the patient require detoxification?
5. What are the patient's prior treatment experiences?
6. What is the current mental status?
7. What is the likelihood of compliance with treatment?
8. What is the potential for acting out?
9. What factors have motivated the patient to seek treatment at this time?
10. What resources and external factors have influenced the patient to seek treatment at this time?

SOURCE: Adapted with permission from Kirstein LS. Inpatient cocaine abuse treatment. Washton AM, Gold MS, eds. *Cocaine: A Clinician's Handbook.* New York: Guilford Publications; 1987:Chap 8.

The route of cocaine administration may determine the extent of physical tests. For example, crack users may require pulmonary function tests; IV drug users may be screened for HIV, hepatitis, and tuberculosis; intranasal users may need ear, nose, and throat evaluation; all patients may require cardiovascular evaluation. In addition, routine laboratory testing should include a:

- Complete blood count (CBC)
- Sequential multiple analysis (SMA)
- Comprehensive and supervised drug screen
- Serum drug screen (when the drug causing a toxicity is unknown)

Qualities of an Inpatient Program

All treatment programs, inpatient or otherwise, should provide supportive therapy that meets the patient's needs. Examples of supportive therapy follow.

- *Medical management* in inpatient programs is often needed either to aid in withdrawal or to treat any coexisting psychiatric or physical illnesses that result from drug abuse. (See Chapter 7 for a discussion of the pharmacotherapy for cocaine abuse.)
- *Family therapy*—essential for success—improves communication among family members. What is more, it develops self-awareness and insight, not just into the patient's problems but the family as a whole.
- *Couples therapy* helps the spouse to deal with

the very difficult issues of codependency and enabling.

- *Group therapy* helps patients gain perspective through contact with other people with similar problems. Group-oriented programs can be quite extensive, encompassing groups such as anonymous groups (AA, CA, and so on); peer support (drug groups, community groups); therapy groups (psychodrama groups, multifamily groups); life skills; and art, dance, or exercise therapies.

- *Individual therapy* is aimed at patients who need special attention for specific problems. For those who are reluctant to participate in group therapy, individual therapy may help to overcome their reluctance.

- *Education* is very much a form of therapy, especially in dealing with substance abusers and their families. Learning the facts about drugs dispels myths and overcomes the rationalizations that perpetuate addiction.

- *Behavioral therapy* focuses on changing the habits associated with addiction and deconditioning responses that could lead to relapse. Relapse prevention (see below) is a behavioral therapy used by more clinicians as the potency of cocaine as a behavioral reinforcer and trigger for relapse has become clear. Other behavioral methods involve aversive conditioning, in which the patient learns to associate negative feelings with drug use. Another behavioral method is to draw up a *contract* that spells out the consequences of behavior—for example, having the patient return to the hospital if he or she is ever caught with drugs. However, behavioral strategies may fail once the patient has left the hospital setting.

- *Exercise programs* and *nutritional counseling* are excellent means of helping addicts regain good health. Most addicts find that their drug use has replaced a healthy diet. As a result, they frequently suffer from nutritional deficiencies that, if left uncorrected, may interfere with their recovery. Other recovery addicts report that a solid exercise regimen reduces the stress of recovery.

- *Compliance monitoring* through urine testing helps patients and treatment providers by supplying an objective means of measuring their abstinence. Most recovering addicts welcome these screens as a valuable aid in their recovery.

- *Workplace liaisons* help to smooth the recovering addict's return to work. This stage of recovery can be very difficult, as both the employer and the recovering employee have many questions. ("How will the other employees treat me?" "What will happen if the employee relapses?" and so on.) A good program should work with the employer and employee to allay these fears. Similarly, a job or career counseling program should be available to help unemployed addicts.

Relapse Prevention

As previously noted, the power of a cocaine high can be so compelling that it can produce overwhelming urges to revert to drug use. Patients whose life-styles revolved around cocaine are susceptible to being reminded of the drug in surprising ways. For example, a patient who sees talcum powder, bread crumbs, or snow may be reminded of cocaine. Seeing cocaine-using friends or locations can trigger drug urges. The click of a cigarette lighter or the light from a match is enough to remind some patients of their cocaine-smoking habit. Apparently, almost any stimulus that has been repeatedly associated with obtaining and using cocaine can become a cocaine "reminder."

Treatment professionals have described a four-step treatment approach to the extinction of cocaine cravings. In the first phase, patients are isolated from the events, subjects, people, and locations that may provoke urges. Next, some of these cues are gradually reintroduced as mental images during psychotherapy sessions. Patients then discuss and rehearse strategies for managing the temptations arising from such provocation. In the third stage, patients reenter their former environments gradually and under the guidance of their caregivers. In the final phase of consolidation, patients continue to participate in self-help and aftercare groups or resume treatment as necessary to counteract any recurring drug cravings.

Relapse prevention strategies using a social learning theory model have been adapted to chemical dependency treatment that follows the disease model.[4] Some of these techniques are: helping the patient recognize the warning signs of relapse; combating the powerful memories of the cocaine euphoria; reinforcing the negative aspects of drugs; overcoming the desire to attempt to regain control over drug use; avoiding the people, places, and things that may trigger drug urges;

preventing occasional "slips" from developing into full-blown binges; learning other ways to cope with unpleasant feelings that in the past may have led to drug use; and developing an array of pleasurable and rewarding alternatives to drugs.

The most promising approach to treatment of cocaine abuse is one that recognizes the high risk of relapse and applies a range of cognitive and behavioral strategies, including a Twelve-Step program, to minimize the risk.

The last ingredient in the recipe for treatment is *follow-up care,* or in the case of inpatient therapy, *discharge planning,* through counseling and continuing access to therapy. As the cessation of inpatient treatment approaches, patients may be granted temporary passes as a means of facilitating their transition to life outside of the hospital. With these passes, patients may return to work, school, and/or family life on a gradual basis. Often, patients who experience cocaine cravings during these passes are relieved to return to the hospital setting where they can confront these cravings and any problems that may have arisen during their time away from the hospital. Relapse prevention strategies can be reinforced during this period.

A discharge planning conference employing all significant members of the patient's rehabilitation team is the final step before discharge. Ideally, this conference will be used to establish an aftercare contract whereby the patient understands the requirements of his or her aftercare and the consequences for violating these policies. Table 6.2 lists the areas that may be covered in a discharge planning session.

It takes incredible stamina and willpower for recovering addicts to remain drug free forever; quite

TABLE 6.2. Discharge Planning Conference

---

1. How long is the term of the contract?
2. What is the frequency of each therapy?
3. What types of therapies will be attended?
4. What is the frequency of anonymous support group meetings?
5. What will be the frequency of urine testing?
6. Will pharmacotherapy be employed, and if so, for how long?
7. Who will be responsible for coordinating the aftercare program?
8. Who can be contacted if there are any deviations from this plan?
9. What are the conditions that would necessitate rehospital-ization?
10. What are the names and phone numbers of contact people?

SOURCE: Adapted with permission from Kirstein LS. Inpatient cocaine abuse treatment. Washton AM, Gold MS, eds. *Cocaine: A Clinician's Handbook*. New York: Guilford Publications; 1987:Chap 8.

understandably, most find it impossible to avoid relapse entirely. Ongoing support through follow-up care is needed to help the patient overcome addiction.

Outcome of Treatment

Relapse among cocaine patients is high; most treatment specialists acknowledge that they offer treatment, not a cure, for addiction. There is reason for hope, however. Perhaps a decade ago, only 10 to 20% of drug addicts recovered following treatment. More recently, a study found that, on average, up to 80% of substance abusers treated for 3 months or longer had reduced their drug use significantly and that 50% were still completely drug free a year after treatment ended.

However, most programs have a high initial drop-out rate, making their data look deceivingly good. Even patients who succeed in treatment with one program may have benefited from previous attempts at treatment with different programs. Furthermore, a treatment program may have a different success rate with various types of drug users. For example, a program that helps a 40-year-old, college-educated executive to recover may not succeed in treating a 19-year-old, unemployed high school dropout. Five-year follow-up data of similar patients, randomly assigned to treatment, are necessary to evaluate treatment success claims. The data results should be confirmed by urine tests.

As in other medical conditions, the results of treatment depend on a variety of factors. Patients whose use of cocaine is low or moderate, who are strongly motivated to become drug free, and who have intact social support networks—family, friends, employers—stand the best chance. People who functioned well before the onset of drug use can usually function well after drug use has ended, provided they remain abstinent and make the necessary changes in life-style. The risk of relapse drops if the patient completes the treatment program and participates in ongoing psychiatric therapy and recovery programs after discharge.

Problems with Cocaine Treatment

An overview on treatment programs published in a 1991 National Institute on Drug Abuse (NIDA) monograph suggested several areas for improving treatment.[5] This overview found that:

- *Too few drug abusers enter treatment.* A recent NIDA survey found that half of all IV drug users have never entered any treatment program. These users, like many drug users, fail to fully understand the benefits of treatment.

- *Addicts in treatment programs continue to abuse drugs.* In a study of an outpatient methadone treatment program, a single drug screen uncovered alarmingly high rates of drug abuse: 26% tested positive for cocaine abuse, and 15% tested positive for opiate (nonmethadone) abuse. This study highlights the importance of using drug screens as an integral part of the treatment process. A recent study of Harvard's inpatient treatment program found drug use common among hospitalized patients.[6] The authors of the study suggested that drug use by one patient often leads to drug use by other patients, perhaps because the initial drug use signaled the availability of drugs and provoked craving in the other patients.
- *Appropriate treatment programs are not matched to the needs of the addict.* Most addicts choose their own treatment program. Neither the addict nor the treatment program attempts to find the treatment program best suited to the addict's needs.
- *Treatment programs ignore the latest medical evidence.* Many treatment programs are mired in the past, continuing to espouse their dated theories without incorporating the latest medical information into their clinical programs.

Treatment for addiction, although difficult and fraught with dangers, can be successful. Millions of recovering addicts are real-life examples of this success. Nevertheless, the best treatment is prevention.

References

1. Gold MS. *The Good News About Drugs and Alcohol.* New York: Villard Books; 1991.
2. Walsh DC, Hingson RW, Merrigan DM, et al. A randomized trial of treatment options for alcohol-abusing workers. *N Eng J Med* 325(11):775–782, 1991.
3. Washton A, Gold MS, Pottash AC. Opiate and cocaine dependencies. *Postgrad Med,* April 1985;77(5):297.
4. Washton A, Gold MS. Cocaine Treatment: A Guide. *American Council for Drug Education.* Rockville, Md., 1986.
5. Pickens RP, Fletcher BW. Overview of Treatment Issues. National Institute on Drug Abuse Research Monograph Series 106: Improving Drug Abuse Treatment; 1991: 1–19.
6. Greenfield SF, Weiss RD, Griffin ML. Patients who use drugs during inpatient substance abuse treatment. *Am J Psychiatry.* 1992;142:235–239.

7

Pharmacological Treatments

At this time, the pharmacological treatments for cocaine addiction are adjunctive and are not intended as
exclusive stand-alone treatments. Rather, their primary
utility stems from helping patients to remain abstinent
and involved in other therapies while coping with the
craving and withdrawal associated with cocaine. Pharmacological treatments may be used for any bona fide
preexisting or concurrent psychiatric conditions. As a
result, these pharmacological treatments can be valuable tools in helping a patient to benefit from the behavioral, rehabilitative, psychotherapeutic, family, and
group therapy (including self-help) treatment regimen
used to promote a successful recovery. Nevertheless,
our increasing knowledge of the physiological effects
of cocaine has led to numerous attempts to improve
and widen the scope of the pharmacotherapy. Table 7.1
lists the most common pharmacological treatments for
cocaine dependence.

TABLE 7.1. Pharmacotherapies for Cocaine Dependence

Antidepressants
Desipramine
Imipramine
Fluoxetine
Sertraline
Bupropion
Dopamine agonists
Bromocriptine
Amantadine
Pergolide
Mazindol
Anticonvulsant
Carbamazepine
Opioid antagonist
Naltrexone
Opioid agonist/antagonist
Buprenorphine
Serotonergic
Ritanserin

In general, research into pharmacological treatments for cocaine-dependent patients has centered on four areas:

1. Cocaine antagonists
2. Drugs that produce an aversive reaction when concomitantly administered with cocaine
3. Psychiatric medications for preexisting disorders
4. Medications that lessen cocaine craving and withdrawal.[1]

Ideally, a *cocaine antagonist* would serve as an effective treatment for acute cocaine toxicity similar to naltrexone's efficacy in treating opioid overdose. Recent research efforts have suggested that the dopamine transporter may be the cocaine receptor. This information, as well as research on cloning of the rat and bovine dopamine transporter and identification of a rapid binding assay for the dopamine transporter,[2] may lead to the development of a pharmacological intervention in cocaine toxicity.

Currently, however, there remains no definitive treatment for cocaine toxicity even though cocaine was the second most common cause of death reported to the American Association of Poison Control Centers in 1988.[3] Numerous treatments, including calcium channel blockers, cold water immersion, antipsychotics, anticonvulsants, and symptomatic support treatments, have been proposed, but further research is necessary, since no solid clinical evidence of their efficacy exists.[1] The anticonvulsant carbamazepine may prove to be an effective pharmacological intervention in cocaine-induced seizures. In animal studies, carbamazepine has been shown to inhibit cocaine-kindled seizures and to improve survival when convulsions were present.[4] Cocaine use may produce stroke, hyperthermia, or arrhythmia, and death following a cocaine-induced seizure may follow immediately. Apparently, the well-publicized deaths of athletes Len Bias and Don Rodgers occurred in this manner.[4] In addition, studies have supported the efficacy of buprenorphine in the treatment of "speedball" (cocaine/opioid mixture) toxicity (see below).

Unlike disulfiram in the treatment of alcohol abuse, no aversive agent for cocaine has been established. However, one uncontrolled study has supported the monoamine oxidase inhibitor (MAOI) phenelzine in the aversive treatment of cocaine abuse.[5] At this time, treatment with phenelzine remains experimental.

Research has supported the efficacy of psychiatric medications in treating the minority of cocaine-dependent patients suffering from comorbid psychiatric disorders, especially when these disorders predate the emergence of drug use. The psychiatric disorders most commonly coexisting with cocaine are major depression, bipolar disorder, cyclothymic disorder, panic disorder, and adult attention deficit disorder. The tricyclic anti-depressant desipramine and lithium have been shown to be effective in the comorbid treatment of depression and bipolar disorders, respectively.[6] (The question of whether desipramine has any benefit for clinically nondepressed patients will be discussed later in the chapter.) Case reports have also supported the use of magnesium pemoline[7] or methylphenidate[8] in cocaine-dependent patients with attention deficit disorder.

Pharmacological Treatment of Cocaine Craving

The pharmacological treatments for cocaine addiction, indeed for all forms of addiction, will likely remain insufficient as long as these treatments focus on withdrawal symptoms and not on the rewarding aspects of drug use. Cravings based on memories of the positive reinforcement of cocaine and further reinforced by the environmental stimuli associated with past drug use create a powerful obstacle to recovery—an obstacle that remains powerful after the temporary discomfort of cocaine withdrawal. Drugs that address only with withdrawal symptoms cannot compete with cocaine craving—hence the high recidivism among cocaine addicts. Wise has stated that "the most effective pharmacological treatment for cocaine craving is cocaine itself."[9]

Understanding the neurochemical disruptions of cocaine may lead to effective pharmacological interventions. Clonidine in the treatment of opiate withdrawal provides an excellent model of this process. The understanding that opiate withdrawal activated noradrenergic hyperactivity suggested that a nonopiate agent that suppressed noradrenergic activity in the locus coeruleus (LC), such as clonidine, would be an effective treatment.[10] Numerous studies of opiate withdrawal and clinical trials have supported this original suggestion. Withdrawal alarm and discomfort may be more universal, since many drugs have increased LC activity associated with withdrawal. Clonidine may be effective in acute cocaine withdrawal as it is for the autonomic component of opiate, alcohol, tranquilizer, and nicotine withdrawal.

In cocaine addiction, the findings that the dopamine system mediates cocaine reward and that chronic cocaine exposure results in DA depletion suggest that DA agents may be effective in the treatment of cocaine addiction.[11] The following sections describe various pharmacological interventions and their effects on the DA system.

Bromocriptine

Several studies have demonstrated the efficacy of the antiparkinsonian medication bromocriptine, a DA receptor agonist, in reducing cocaine cravings.[12] Bromocriptine reverses the cocaine-induced changes in

DA receptor supersensitivity, DA depletion, and hyperprolactinemia. The anticraving efficacy of bromocriptine has been supported by both open and double-blind placebo-controlled studies.[13,14] Preliminary results of a recent study of inpatients being treated for cocaine withdrawal found that both bromocriptine and pergolide significantly reduced craving while increasing mean length of stay when compared to a group receiving no medication (see Figure 7.1).[15] While finding that bromocriptine worked against craving, Tennant and Sagherian also reported significant side effects (including nausea, headaches, and orthostatic hypotension)

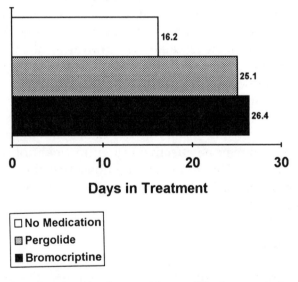

FIGURE 7.1. Mean length of stay with pergolide, bromocriptine, and no medication. SOURCE: Malcolm R. Pergolide, bromocriptine trial in cocaine addiction. Am Psychiatric Assoc; 1992. Abstract NR:332.

with doses totaling 15 mg daily.[16] Our experience has been that total daily doses of 2–10 mg prove effective without incurring significant side effects (see Table 7.2). The optimum length of the bromocriptine trial has not been fully established; it may be necessary to reinstate therapy if cravings recur following discontinuation.

We have previously hypothesized that while acute cocaine administration produces a temporary dopamine increase, repeated administration produces an absolute decrease in dopamine that can be temporally corrected by another cocaine administration.[17,18] The cycle of depletion, cocaine administration, and further depletion may be what is seen in laboratory animals and human beings as cocaine binges and relapse. If cocaine abstinence is associated with an absolute or relative depletion of dopamine, then medications that increase

TABLE 7.2. Bromocriptine Protocol

Day	Dose (mg)	Frequency
1–2	1.25	b.i.d.
3–4	1.25	t.i.d.
5–6	2.5	b.i.d.
7–11	2.5	t.i.d.
12–14	5	b.i.d.
15–20	Decrease by 50% every 2 days	

Note: Titration of the dose is necessary with anticraving and antiwithdrawal effects weighed against side effects. Lower doses than listed above are often sufficient. Maintenance bromocriptine treatment may be necessary if symptoms recur when discontinuation is attempted.
SOURCE: Reprinted with permission from Dackis CA, Gold MS. Treatment strategies for cocaine detoxification. In Lakowski JM, Galloway MP, White FP, eds. *Pharmacology, Physiology, and Clinical Strategies.* Boca Raton, Fla.: CRC Press; 1992:421:chap 19.

functional dopamine by mimicking dopamine or that increase the absolute amount of dopamine available at the synapse should be therapeutically useful.

To test this hypothesis directly and compare the efficacy of the two main treatments for acute cocaine abstinence-related dysphoria and depression, we administered desipramine (DMI) and bromocriptine (BROMO) to 12 young adults (three women and nine men). These individuals were chronic cocaine crack smokers who met DSM-III-R criteria for cocaine dependence and who complained of clinically significant "withdrawal" symptoms. All were studied within 72 hours of acute admission to a locked hospital ward after giving written informed consent for oral administration of a single dose of bromocriptine (1.25 mg) and desipramine (50 mg) on consecutive days. The study used a double-blind random assignment crossover design. Craving, mood, and energy were self-rated before and 1, 3, 6, 8, and 12 hours after each medication. Although variability was high, baseline symptoms before BROMO and before DMI did not differ significantly. At six hours, BROMO reduced mean craving 48% ($p < 0.05$, paired t test), lessened depressed mood 38% ($p < 0.10$), and increased energy by 21% ($p < 0.05$). DMI reduced craving 41% ($p < 0.01$), reduced energy 19% ($p < 0.01$), and had no effect on mood. In patients with high pretreatment symptomatology, both medications reduced craving ($p < 0.05$), but only BROMO lessened depressed mood and increased energy ($p < 0.05$). Reports of side effects were not specific to either medication.

Amantadine, another dopamine agonist, has also been shown to reduce cocaine craving. Amantadine and bromocriptine both release DA into the synapse.

This supports a DA theory for cocaine withdrawal dysphoria but also has led some theorists to suggest that they may "prime" the user for cocaine and eventually result in renewed cravings for cocaine when the effects of the medication wear off.[9] However, numerous studies have supported the anticraving and treatment benefits of both medications, suggesting that the amount of DA released is sufficient to alleviate craving without inducing relapse. Eventually, pharmacotherapy with DA agonists may allow the dopaminergic system to achieve homeostasis in a cocaine-free environment.

Tricyclic Antidepressants (TCAs)

Interestingly, TCAs block DA and NE reuptake while increasing postsynaptic DA sensitivity,[19] effects that are similar to those achieved by cocaine (see Table 7.3). Some studies of outpatients treated with desipramine and imipramine have supported the anticraving and treatment benefits of TCAs.[20] However, Weiss and colleagues reported that desipramine was associated with higher rates of recidivism.[21] Furthermore, recent studies by Kosten et al. (1992)[22] and Arndt et al. (1992)[23] have failed to substantiate the benefits of TCA therapy. In fact, Arndt et al. (1992) found that placebo-treated subjects improved during the 6-month period following treatment, while desipramine-receiving group continued to show a high level of cocaine use. Other studies have failed to find any treatment benefit, suggesting that any efficacy associated with TCAs derives from their effect upon coexisting affective illness,[12] or

TABLE 7.3. Antidepressant Effects on Dopamine and
Norepinephrine Uptake[24]

Antidepressant	Dopamine uptake block	Norepinephrine uptake block
Amitriptyline	+1	+2
Amoxapine	+1	+3
Bupropion	+2	+/−
Desipramine	+/−	+4
Doxepin	+/−	+2
Fluoxetine	+1	+1
Imipramine	+/−	+2
Maprotiline	+1	+3
Nortriptyline	+1	+3
Protriptyline	+1	+4
Sertaline	+3	+1
Trazodone	0	+/−
Trimipramine	+1	+1

Potency: +4 = most potent   +/− = weak effect   0 = no effect

possibly from their use with specific populations of outpatients.[25]

Other antidepressants, including fluoxetine and bupropion (a bicyclic antidepressant with prolactin lowering and predominantly DA activity), have been tried in the treatment of cocaine abuse. In fact, preliminary studies with bupropion have been associated with abstinence rates of 70%.[26]

Carbamazepine

The rationale for pharmacotherapy with carbamazepine derives from the hypothesis that craving may be the behavioral manifestation of "kindling," the progressive neuronal firing in discrete regions of the brain that can result in animals after repeated exposure to cocaine (see Chapter 3). In animals, the anticonvulsant carbamazepine inhibits the early stages of kindling caused by local anesthetics,[27] and significantly prevents cocaine-induced seizures while inhibiting the lethality associated with cocaine-induced convulsions.[4] Preliminary results from a study of 16 crack cocaine addicts found that carbamazepine compliance was associated with successful abstinence.[28] Although these results are promising, controlled clinical trials are necessary.

Buprenorphine

Recently, buprenorphine, the opioid mixed agonist-antagonist that has some methadonelike effects and some naltrexonelike effects, has been tried in the treatment of cocaine- and opioid-abusing outpatients.[29] Buprenorphine appears to combine the patient acceptance and cross-tolerance that make the agonist methadone clinically effective as a maintenance treatment with the narcotic blocking ability of naltrexone. In addition, little physical dependence has been shown for buprenorphine. Doses of 4 to 8 mg per day of buprenorphine are adequate for opiate blockade and appear to block the effects of cocaine.[30] Kosten and coworkers recently reported comparison of buprenorphine to methadone in 130 opioid-dependent patients who also used cocaine and found that buprenorphine had better efficacy than 65 mg of methadone per day.[31] Furthermore, in animals, buprenorphine produced a dose-dependent protection against the lethal effects of cocaine.[30] The ultimate abuse potential of buprenorphine will be determined in the ongoing clinical trials, but Cone and coworkers have recently reported long-acting behavioral effects and abuse liability of intravenous buprenorphine.[32] Animal studies have suggested a possible benefit in decreased cocaine craving;[33] however, the question of buprenorphine's abuse potential remains.

Naltrexone

The opiate antagonist naltrexone may prove to attenuate cocaine self-administration. Our clinical experience with physician addicts supports this view, since naltrexone compliance was associated with abstinence from opiates *and* cocaine.[34] While the dopaminergic system has been viewed by many as the most essential factor in cocaine reinforcement, other systems, including serotonergic and opioid systems, may also be involved. Opioid systems have been implicated in the reinforcement of a number of abused drugs (such as opiates and alcohol), and opioid involvement has been shown in a number of reports on cocaine self-administration.[35] A study by Ramsey and van Ree found that naltrexone significantly attenuated cocaine self-administration in rats, supporting the involvement of opioid systems in cocaine reinforcement and suggesting that effects of naltrexone opiate agonists lessen cocaine reinforcement.[35] Additional studies are required before naltrexone's efficacy in limiting cocaine reinforcement in human beings can be determined.

Volpicelli et al. (1992) reported that naltrexone decreased alcohol craving, mean drinking days, and relapse rates in 70 alcohol dependent males.[36] The authors reported that naltrexone seemed especially beneficial in decreasing drinking in patients who had at least one previous "slip." This study supports the hypothesis that at least some part of alcohol's reinforcement stems from opioid involvement.

Miscellaneous Agents

Sulpiride is a selective D2 receptor blocker with antipsychotic and antidepressant effects. Currently marketed in Europe, sulpiride has been shown to inhibit cocaine-induced defensive behavior, suggesting that the hyperdefensiveness of chronic cocaine abusers may be produced by changes in D2 receptor functioning.[37] Previous studies have also shown that self-administration of cocaine could be attenuated by sulpiride in rats.[38]

The ability of neuroleptics to block the euphoric effects of amphetamine has been known for several years, but their use in abstinent cocaine users has been associated with increased craving.[39] This finding, combined with the apparent sensitivity of cocaine addicts to neuroleptic side effects and the risk of tardive dyskinesia, suggests that neuroleptic therapy in cocaine recovery is very problematic.

Ritanserin, a serotonin 5-HT_2 antagonist, has been found to reduce cocaine consumption among rats.[40] This finding suggests the importance of the serotonin in addition to DA in cocaine addiction, and also suggests that ritanserin may interfere with the mechanisms responsible for the reinforcement that occurs after repeated exposure to cocaine.

While the search for safer and more effective pharmacological interventions continues, one should realize that it is extremely unlikely that any nonaddicting medication will ever match the addictive and reinforcing power of cocaine. In addition, the rewarding properties associated with nonaddicting, anticraving medications will probably never equal the memories associated with the reinforcing properties of cocaine. As a result, the problem of relapse will inevitably continue to plague the treatment of cocaine addiction. Therefore, the most effective treatment for cocaine addiction remains prevention: In the absence of use, cocaine addiction simply cannot develop.

References

1. Weiss RD, Mirin SM. Psychological and pharmacological treatment strategies in cocaine dependence. *Ann Clin Psychiatry.* 1990;2:239–243.
2. Vaughan RA, Simantov R, Lew R, Kuhar MJ. A rapid binding assay for solubilized dopamine transporters using [^{3}H]WIN 35,428. *J Neurosci Methods.* 1991;40:9–16.
3. Goldfrank LR, Hoffman RS. American Association of Poison Control Centers National Data Collection System. *Ann Emerg Med.* 1991;20:165–170.
4. Post RM, Weiss SRB, Aigner TC. Carbamazepine in the treatment of cocaine abuse. Paper presented at the Conference on the Biological Basis of Addiction; Santa Monica, Calif; January 11, 1991.
5. Golwyn DH. Cocaine abuse treated with phenelzine. *Int J Addict.* 1988;23:897–905.
6. Gawin FH, Kleber HD, Byck R, et al. Desipramine facilitation of initial cocaine abstinence. *Arch Gen Psychiatry.* 1989;46:117–121.
7. Weiss RD, Pope HG Jr, Mirin SM. Treatment of chronic abuse and attention deficit disorder, residual type, with magnesium pemoline. *Drug Alcohol Depend.* 1985;15:69–72.
8. Khantzian EJ. An extreme case of cocaine dependence and marked improvement with methylphenidate treatment. *Am J Psychiatry.* 1983;140:784–785.

9. Wise RA. The neurobiology of craving: implications for the understanding and treatment of addiction. *J Abnormal Psychol.* 1988;97(2)118–132.
10. Gold MS, Pottash ALC, Extein I, et al. Clonidine in acute opiate withdrawal. *N Eng J Med.* 1980;302:1421.
11. Dackis CA, Gold MS. Pharmacological approaches to cocaine addiction. *J Substance Abuse Treatment.* 1985;2:139.
12. Dackis CA, Gold MS. Treatment strategies for cocaine detoxification. Lakowski JM, Galloway MP, White FP, eds. In *Cocaine: Pharmacology, Physiology, and Clinical Strategies.* Boca Raton, Fla: CRC Press; 1992: Chap 19.
13. Extein IL, Gross DA, Gold MS. Cocaine detoxification using bromocriptine. *Am Psychiatric Assoc;* 1986. Abstract NR 70.
14. Giannini AJ, Baumgartel P, Dimarzio LR. Bromocriptine therapy in cocaine withdrawal. *J Clin Pharmacol.* 1987;27:267.
15. Malcolm R. Pergolide, bromocriptine trial in cocaine addiction. *Am Psychiatric Assoc;* 1992. Abstract NR:332.
16. Tennant FS, Sagherian AA. Double-blind comparison of amantadine hydrochloride and bromocriptine mesylate for ambulatory withdrawal from cocaine dependence. *Arch Intern Med.* 1987;147:109.
17. Gold MS, Dackis CA. New insights and treatments: opiate withdrawal and cocaine addiction. *Clin Ther.* 1984;7:6–21.
18. Dackis CA, Gold MS. New concepts in cocaine addiction: the dopamine depletion hypothesis. *Neurosci Biobehav Rev.* 1985;9: 469–477.
19. Spyraki C, Fibinger HC. Behavioral evidence for supersensitivity of postsynaptic dopamine receptors in the mesolimbic system after chronic administration of desipramine. *Eur J Pharmacol.* 1981;74:195.
20. Gawin FH. Cocaine addiction: psychology and neurophysiology. *Science.* 1991;251:1580–1585.
21. Weiss RD, Mirin SM, and Michael JL. Relapse to cocaine abuse after initiating desipramine treatment. *JAMA.* 1988;260:2545.
22. Kosten TR, Morgan CM, Falcione J, Schotenfeld RS. Pharmacotherapy for cocaine abusing methadone maintained patients using amantadine or desipramine. *Arch Gen Psychiatry* 49:904-908, 1992.
23. Arndt IO, Dorozynsky L, Woody GE, McLellan AT, O'Brien CP.

Desipramine treatment of cocaine dependence in methadone maintenance patients. *Arch Gen Psychiatry* 49:904-908, 1992.

24. *Pharmacological Effects of Antidepressants,* Version II Physicians Postgraduate Press, Inc; 1992.

25. Meyer RE. New pharmacotherapies for cocaine dependence . . . revisited. *Arch Gen Psychiatry* 49:900-904, 1992.

26. Kosten TR. Behavioral and pharmacologic treatments for cocaine dependence. Treatment challenges in the 1990s. Washington, DC: American Psychiatric Association; May 1992.

27. Post RM. Time course of clinical effects of carbamazepine: implication for mechanism of action. *J Clin Psychiatry.* 1988;49(suppl) 4(1):35–46.

28. Halikas JA, Kuhn KL, Crea FS, et al. Treatment of crack cocaine use with carbamazepine. *Am J Drug Alcohol Abuse.* 1992;18(1): 45–56.

29. Gastfriend DR, Mendelson JH, Mello NK, Teoh SK. Preliminary results of an open trial of buprenorphine in the outpatient treatment of combined heroin and cocaine dependence. Committee on Problems of Drug Dependence, 53rd Annual Scientific Meeting; Palm Beach, Fla; June 16–20, 1991.

30. Grayson NA, Witkin JM, Katz JL, Cowan A, Rice KC. Actions of buprenorphine of cocaine and opiate mediated effects. Committee on Problems of Drug Dependence, 53rd Annual Scientific Meeting; Palm Beach, Fla; June 16–20, 1991.

31. Kosten TR, Schottenfeld RS, Morgan C, Falcioni J, Ziedonis D. Buprenorphine vs. methadone for opioid and cocaine dependence. Committee on Problems of Drug Dependence, 53rd Annual Scientific Meeting; Palm Beach, Fla; June 16–20, 1991.

32. Cone E, Holicky B, Pickworth W, Johnson RE. Pharmacologic and behavioral effects of high doses of intravenous buprenorphine. Committee on Problems of Drug Dependence, 53rd Annual Scientific Meeting; Palm Beach, Fla; June 16–20, 1991.

33. Kosten TR. Behavioral and pharmacologic treatments for cocaine dependence. American Psychiatric Association Symposium: Treatment Challenges in the 1990s. May 1992. Washington, D.C.

34. Washton AM, Pottash ALC, Gold MS. Naltrexone in addicted business executives and physicians. *J Clin Psychiatry.* 1984;45(9): 39–41.

35. Ramsey NF, van Ree JM. Intracerebroventricular naltrexone

treatment attenuates acquisition of intravenous cocaine self-administration in rats. *Pharm Biochem Behav.* 1991;40:807–810.

36. Volpicelli JR, Berg BJ, Alterman AI, et al. Naltrexone in the treatment of alcohol dependence. New Research #331, American Psychiatric Association Annual Meeting, Washington DC, May 1992.

37. Filibeck U, Cabib S, Castellana C, Puglisi-Allegra S. Chronic cocaine enhances defensive behaviors in the laboratory mouse: involvement of the D2 dopamine receptors. *Psychopharmacology.* 1988;96:437–441.

38. Goeders NE, Smith JE. Cortical dopaminergic involvement in cocaine reinforcement. *Science.* 1983; 221(4612):773–775.

39. Daekis CA, Gold MS, Davies RK, Sweeney DR. Bromocriptine treatment for cocaine abuse: the dopamine depletion hypothesis. *Int J Psychiatry Med.* 1985;15:125.

40. Meert TF, Janssen PA. Ritanserin, a new therapeutic approach for drug abuse. Part 2: effects on cocaine. *Drug Develop Res.* 1992;25:39–53.

8

The Role of Drug Testing

Perhaps the most controversial drug-related issue to originate in the 1980s concerned drug testing. In 1982, a National Institute on Drug Abuse booklet on employee drug abuse failed to even mention the subject of drug screens; by 1990, over 60% of 1000 companies conducted some form of employee drug testing.[1] This increase in drug testing emanated from an increasing awareness of the deleterious effects that drug use inflicts on businesses in the form of increased health care costs, greater safety risks, increased employee theft, and decreased productivity. Consider the following:

- As many as 65% of the young people entering the work force have used illegal drugs.[2]
- The National Institute on Drug Abuse (NIDA) estimates that one out of eight workers between the ages of 26 and 35 abuse drugs, including alcohol, while at work.[3]

- For younger workers aged 18 and 25, the numbers are even higher: 20% use drugs on the job.[3]
- Drug users incur medical costs that on average are *three times as high* as the rest of a company's employees.
- Drug users are absent from work twice as often as nonusing employees.[4]
- Users are five times as likely to be involved in accidents when off the job.[4]
- Contrary to the beliefs of many people, the majority of drug users are employed (see Figure 8.1).

One of the biggest factors behind the rise of drug education and drug testing was the Drug Free Workplace Act of 1988. This federal legislation requires all companies to certify themselves as providing a drug-free workplace if they receive government grants or if they buy property or services worth more than $25,000 from any federal agency.[5]

We have already begun to see the positive effects of increased attention directed toward drug abuse. In 1990, SmithKline Beckman reported that 13% of their 1 million workers and job applicants tested positive for drug abuse during the first 6 months of 1990. This finding, although still significant, represents a dramatic decline from 1987, when 18% tested positive. The president of the company attributed this decline to greater attention to drug abuse in the workplace.[1]

It is ironic that, while drug testing has become a common practice in business, the medical profession has been relatively slow to implement the practice. Few physicians routinely order diagnostic drug screens, even in patients with a high risk of drug abuse. The

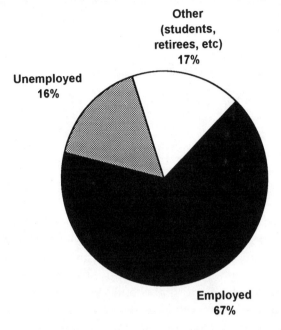

FIGURE 8.1. Employment status of current adult drug users, 1991.
SOURCE: NIDA National Household Survey, 1991.

DSM-III-R does not discuss even their diagnostic utility. Medical schools rarely screen their students for
drug use, even though studies indicate a high rate of
drug abuse among medical students (see Chapter 10).
A recent study of 1088 women undergoing their first
prenatal examination found that 166 (15.26%) tested
positive for drug use. Forty percent of those testing
positive denied any drug use; the researchers concluded
that the routine screening of populations at risk for drug
abuse should be considered.[6] It is hoped that drug

screens will soon become widely accepted as a diagnostic and preventive measure in the medical profession.

The Evolution of Drug Testing

Since the 1960s, emergency room physicians have used drug tests to assist in the diagnosis and treatment of patients who are comatose, overdosed, or intoxicated. In the late 1970s, physicians began using drug tests to help in the psychiatric evaluation of prospective patients. Drug tests could indicate to the physician whether a "manic" patient was really manic or using stimulants. However, in industry, the idea of screening urine or blood samples for evidence of drug use is relatively new. Drug testing emerged as a viable business strategy when the technology became sophisticated enough to assure that results were accurate, and simple enough for medical technicians to perform without years of training. These developments have occurred only within the last 10 years. The Greyhound Corporation is generally credited with pioneering the drug-testing movement in the early 1980s. After they launched their program, other companies, including American Airlines, IBM, Burlington Northern Railroad, Georgia Power Company, Southern Pacific, General Motors, and Exxon followed suit.[5]

Although somewhat controversial, drug testing is gaining widespread acceptance in both the public and private sectors. In a survey of adult workers across the country, over 97% said that some form of drug testing at work is appropriate under certain circumstances. More than 9 out of 10 thought it was a good idea to test pilots and truck drivers.[7]

Whatever the financial and legal reasons behind it, drug testing—used properly and fairly and with regard for the individual's civil rights—can identify drug users and trigger a successful intervention. The earlier the intervention, the greater the chance that treatment will be successful.[8] Similarly, treatment programs can use regular drug screens either to verify objectively a patient's abstinence or to identify relapses.

Another benefit of testing is that it acts as a deterrent. For example, before the Coast Guard began testing personnel for drugs, as many as 1 out of 10 members used drugs. Now that testing is routine, less than 2% use drugs. The Federal Aviation Administration found even lower rates; only about one half of 1% of employees in random tests were found to be drug abusers.[1]

The "Demographics" of Drug Testing

Businesses most likely to have testing programs are the mining industry, including oil and gas facilities; communications and public utilities; and transportation. As I've noted, some of these companies test in order to comply with regulatory requirements. The least likely to test are retailers, construction companies, and the service industries. One reason is that such companies are more likely to have fewer than 10 employees, and they usually have a high turnover rate.[9] Widespread testing by the military produced an 82% drop in drug use since 1981.[10]

Of those businesses with testing programs, 85% test new job applicants (preemployment testing) and 64% focus on current employees (random or annual testing). Most of them test all applicants before offering the applicants a position. Only 16% limited testing to people applying for specific jobs within a company. In those companies that test their employees, two out of three do so only when they suspect a problem with drugs, but one in four tests everybody. In 1 year, roughly 9 workers out of 100 who work for companies with drug-testing programs—a total of nearly a million people—were actually asked to submit to tests.[9] Of these, about 9% tested positive. Of the 3.9 million job applicants who submitted to tests, 12% tested positive.

A recent study of 4396 U.S. postal workers hired regardless of the results of a preemployment drug screen found that 9% tested positive for illegal drugs (see Figure 8.2).[11] Over a period of 15 months, the absenteeism rates, injuries, accidents, and job turnover rates of these employees were tracked. The study found that those who tested positive for drug use were nearly twice as likely to be absent from work and were one and a half times more likely to be fired. The authors of the study estimated that hiring these drug-positive employees cost the Postal Service $4 million in lost productivity in 1 year and almost $53 million over their full employment tenure.

The federal Department of Transportation (DOT) began testing all of its employees in 1988, a move that initially affected 32,000 workers, mostly air traffic controllers. Starting in late 1989 and continuing through 1990, the department also implemented testing policies that covered nearly 4 million workers, including aviation personnel, interstate truck drivers, maritime shippers and seamen, railroad workers, employees of companies operating gas pipelines, and urban mass transit workers.

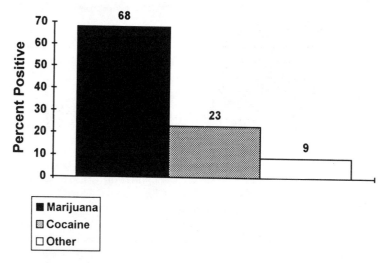

FIGURE 8.2. Breakdown of drug screens of U.S. postal employees. SOURCE: Normad J, Salyards SD, Mahoney JJ. An evaluation of preemployment drug testing. U.S. Postal Service, Washington, DC. American Psychological Association Press Release; December 1990.

In October 1991, President Bush signed legislation that extended the DOT testing policies to mass transit employees and intrastate truckers, bringing the total number of workers covered by DOT policies to approximately 6 million.[12] The DOT program calls for random testing of employees in safety-related jobs, as well as testing before employment, after accidents, when drug use is suspected, and at fixed times, such as during routine medical exams. Figure 8.3 illustrates the positive effects of the DOT testing program.

Other government agencies are following suit. The Nuclear Regulatory Commission implemented testing rules in 1989, and recently the Department of Defense

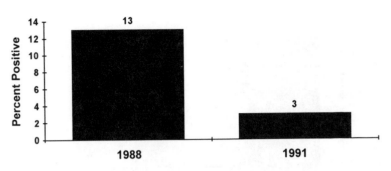

FIGURE 8.3. Positive drug screens for transportation workers before and after drug-testing program. SOURCE: National Drug Control Strategy, the White House; January 1992:50.

demanded that all of its contractors with access to classified information must set up and maintain drug-free workplaces.[5]

IBM's approach is often cited as a model for others to follow. IBM tests all job applicants; if results are positive, they must wait 6 months before they can reapply. If an employee shows a decline in performance, is absent for prolonged periods for unexplained reasons, or shows other erratic behavior, the supervisor reports the problem to the medical department. The employee meets with the company physician and submits to an evaluation, including, perhaps, a drug test. Some IBM jobs are considered "safety-sensitive"; people in these positions must agree to undergo a test or they will be fired. If test results are positive, the employee enters the assistance program. Before returning to work the employee must be drug free, take part in a rehabilitation or treatment program, and agree to be monitored by the physician, including periodic, un-scheduled urine testing.[10]

The majority of drug-testing programs currently use urine samples, with blood samples used primarily to measure very recent cocaine use and its effect on behavior. However, new methods of detecting substance abuse, using less invasive techniques than urine or blood analysis, are currently being investigated. Drug screens using hair or saliva may someday become commonplace. In fact, one study of saliva in cocaine users suggests that saliva may be more sensitive than urinalysis.[13]

The Most Common Forms of Urinalysis

Drug testing should be a two-step process. The recommended testing protocols use an initial screen to identify positive samples. Any positive screen must be confirmed by another test that is more specific and reliable than the screening test.

In general, screening tests may be divided into two categories: (1) immunoassays (enzyme immunoassays and radioimmunoassays) and (2) chromatographic (thin layer chromatography [TLC]).

Immunoassay Screens

The enzyme immunoassay (EIA) and the radio-immunoassay (RIA) tests use antibodies to attach to drugs that may be present in the urine test mixture. In the EIA, the interaction of the antibodies with the drug causes a color change that can be measured by a spectrophotometer. In the RIA test, this interaction results in emission of a low level of radiation. This radiation is then measured by a gamma counter. Because of this radiation, the RIA may be performed only in the licensed facility by specially trained technicians. However, the EIA may be used in a laboratory, in a physician's office, or even at the workplace. Both the EIA and the RIA are designed to detect amphetamines, barbiturates, benzodiazepines, marijuana, cocaine, methaqualone, opiates, and phencyclidine.

Both EIA and RIA have the potential problem of *cross-reactivity*. Substances whose chemical structures are similar to the drug that is being screened for may cross-react with antibodies used in immunoassays and cause false-positives. Media reports have focused on nonprescription medication appearing as amphetamines, ibuprofen being identified as marijuana, and antibiotics appearing as cocaine. The possibility of cross-reactivity makes absolutely necessary the confirmation of all positives by a more accurate and different test.

The accuracy of EIA screens is approximately 95%. The 5% error rate results primarily from false-negatives, where the person who is using drugs is not identified.[14]

Also, individuals may tamper with their urine specimen by adding adulterants such as lemon juice and vinegar (acidic liquids), chlorine bleach and other caustics (alkaline liquids), and sodium chloride (salt). These adulterants may cause false-negatives. To identify samples that may be tampered with, the lab should also check for *pH* and *specific gravity levels*.

The RIA test works in a similar way to EIA tests, but the RIA equipment is more complex, and extensive training is required. It may be preferable to use RIA when handling large numbers of samples, since the test is more compatible with the automated equipment necessary for high volume.

The EIA and RIA both have the advantage of giving definitive results with no need for interpretation by a technician. These tests are more sensitive and can detect more minute amounts of a drug than can thin layer chromatography. Conversely, both RIA and EIA are more expensive than TLC and do not detect as many drugs as does TLC.

Chromatographic Screens

The most common chromatographic drug screen is thin layer chromatography. TLC involves removing the liquid portion of the urine and chemically treating the residue to separate its various chemical compounds. A dye solution, sprayed on the urine sample, causes color changes. Individual drugs are then identified visually, depending on their color and location in the sample. TLC can test for up to 40 drugs in one sample.

Compared to EIA/RIA, TLC has the advantages of being less expensive while allowing screening for a greater number of drugs. However, its biggest disadvantage is that technicians must use their judgment in interpreting the results. A number of substances in the urine sample may interfere and cause spots that can easily be identified as a positive result. A high degree of technical expertise is required, making TLC vulnerable to questions and to errors in judgment. What appears to be yellow may not appear that way to another technician. In addition, the dye used in TLC fades quickly—there is no permanent record of the test *unless a photograph is taken.* This means that TLC results may be less likely to stand up to a legal challenge.

Also, TLC is not as sensitive as EIA/RIA. Frequently, TLC requires that the minimum amount of a drug or drug by-product necessary to yield a positive result falls between 1000 and 2000 ng/mL (as compared to a low of 20 ng/mL for EIA). Although TLC screens are still widely used, the immunoassays are gaining precedence in industrial screening programs.

Regardless of whether the testing protocol relies on TLC or EIA/RIA for its initial screen, confirmation of all positive screens must be made.

Confirmation Tests

Although gas chromatography (GC) is sometimes used alone as a confirmation test, the most accurate method combines it with mass spectrometry. In GC, the liquid sample undergoes heating and vaporizing as it passes through a column of absorbent material. Individual compounds are separated and identified on this column according to their chemical and physical properties. These separated compounds will then appear as peaks to the GC detector.

Gas chromatography/mass spectrometry (GC/MS) uses gas chromatography combined with a mass spectrometer to produce a test that is currently the most accurate test available. GC/MS continues to break down the individual compounds identified by gas chromatography into electrically charged ion fragments. Every compound has a specific ion structure, with no two structures the same. These ion fragments that are isolated by GC/MS have a specific pattern that can be positively identified with the pattern for known drugs of abuse. GC/MS, when properly conducted, is extremely accurate.[1]

This test requires highly trained technicians and expensive equipment. The high cost makes GC/MS too prohibitive to be used as a mass screening instrument. But it is the best and most reliable means of confirming initial positive tests.

Evaluation of Testing Facilities

The National Institute on Drug Abuse has developed a set of rigid standards a laboratory must meet before it will be allowed to conduct drug tests on government employees. These guidelines cover every possible aspect of the test, from acquisition to storage, to analysis, to the final report. A chain of custody must be established to assure that the sample never falls into unauthorized hands. Mistakes can still occur, but NIDA has established strict standards to minimize their occurrence. So demanding are these standards that only 33 out of more than 200 laboratories earned the NIDA seal of approval.[15]

Companies have the responsibility to make sure their drug-testing protocols respect individual rights while guaranteeing the highest degree of accuracy possible. Protocols must consider worker's rights, including the right to privacy. Drug testing should not be considered as a weapon but as a means of early detection and deterrence and as an extremely valuable tool to aid in a patient's recovery.

The following discussion with Mark A. de Bernardo, one of this country's top legal experts on drug testing, explains some of the pitfalls that companies may face.

*What **Not** to Do: Common Employer Mistakes in Addressing Drug Abuse: A Discussion with Mark A. de Bernardo, Executive Director of the Institute for a Drug-Free Workplace and Resident Partner in the Washington, DC Law Office of Littler, Medelson, Fastiff and Tichy*

Q: *Should a drug abuse policy address alcohol abuse?*
A: Alcohol remains the most commonly abused drug in America—and in American workplaces. It is clear that in many ways illicit drug abuse compromises the workplace more substantially (stealing, dealing, violence, ties to organized crime) than alcohol abuse and, to a certain extent, drug abuse is harder to detect. Nonetheless, the virtually identical psychology of addition, the comparable safety risks and decreased productivity, and the increased incidence of polydrug abuse (alcohol and illicit drugs) make alcohol a critical threat to employers and employees and warrants parallel company programs to address alcohol and drug problems. You do not have a drug-free workplace if you tolerate excessive alcohol use.

Q: *What should a supervisor or manager do when confronting suspected drug users?*
A: Supervisors and managers should be cautioned never to take action alone against someone suspected of dealing or using drugs on the job, or being "under the influence." First of all, to do so could be physically dangerous. Second, there is substantial legal value to having a reliable witness or witnesses present in the event of a subsequent legal challenge.

Also, a supervisor should not send the employee home behind the steering wheel of a car. By the same token, to restrain the employee from leaving—taking him or her in custody—could subject the employer to claims of false imprisonment. What should an employer do? After other appropriate actions under the company policy (e.g., a drug test, conditional suspension), the employer should either call a cab for the employee or, more appropriately, have a supervisor or coworker drive him or her home.

Q. *What happens if an employer inconsistently enforces its drug policy?*
A. To do so is an invitation to litigation. Like most areas of

labor and employment law, employers have great latitude in what their policies on drug abuse are going to be. However, once that policy is adopted, an employer must adhere to it. This means taking the *same action* in response to a policy violation for senior or highly valued employees as for newly hired or very marginal employees. If you repeatedly treat similar violations for company policy differently, ultimately you will be sued and you will lose.

This policy, by the way, must be written and well-communicated to employees. Never take enforcement action based simply on spoken or "understood" rules . . . the legal consequences can be highly detrimental. Given the costs of litigation when you as an employer go to court, even if you win . . . you lose.

Q. *Should an employer implement a "fitness for duty" policy?*
A. When an employer prohibits drug use that renders an employee "unfit for duty," or "under the influence," that employer is needlessly backing itself in a corner. Performance-related standards are subject to interpretation—and litigation. Forget performance standards. Prohibit illicit drug use . . . period. You should not care if the drug use took place on break time in the company parking lot, before work outside the factory gates, or the night before at the employee's home. A confirmed "positive" drug test demonstrates the presence of illicit drugs, and that in and of itself should be a violation of company policy sufficient to trigger adverse employment action.

Q. *How important is the confidentiality of drug test results?*
A. Only those with a "need to know" should be informed of the results of an employee drug test. More widely disseminated test results may trigger tort actions against the employer for, among other claims, defamation, invasion of privacy, intentional infliction of emotional distress, and/or negligent infliction of emotional distress. Legal considerations aside, it simply is good employee relations to strive to minimize any unwarranted intrusions into employees' privacy.

Source: Adapted with permission from MS Gold (Ed.), The University of Florida's *Facts About Drugs and Alcohol Newsletter* 2(1): Winter 1993.

References

1. Gold MS. *The Good News About Drugs and Alcohol.* New York: Villard Books, 1991.
2. Watkins GT. Window of opportunity. *EAP Dig.* September/October 1989:6.
3. Feingold BC. Deterring damage. *Employee Assist.* October 1989; 2(3):29–30.
4. Freudenheim M. More aid for addicts on the job. *New York Times.* November 13, 1989.
5. Appel CB. A winning team. *Employee Assist.* October 1989;2(3): 23–25.
6. Colmorgen GHC, Johnson C, Zazzarine MA, Durinzi K. Routine urine drug screening at the first prenatal visit. *Am J Obstet Gynecol.* 1992;166:588–590.
7. Cushman JH Jr. Private transportation workers to join ranks of those tested for drug use. *New York Times.* December 18, 1989;D9.
8. Verebey K, Gold MS, Mulé SJ. Laboratory testing in the diagnosis of marijuana intoxication and withdrawal. *Psychiatric Ann.* April 1986;16(4):235–241.
9. U.S. Department of Labor, Bureau of Labor Statistics. Survey of Employer Anti-Drug Programs. U.S. Department of Labor Report 760; January 1989.
10. The White House. National Drug Control Strategy, Office of National Drug Control Policy; September 1989.
11. Normad J, Salyards SD, Mahoney JJ. An evaluation of preemployment drug testing. U.S. Postal Service, Washington, DC. American Psychological Association Press Release; December 1990.
12. The White House National Drug Control Strategy, Office of National Drug Control Policy; January 1992.
13. Increased chances of cocaine detection with saliva testing. *Forensic Drug Abuse Advisor.* May 1992;4(5):37.
14. Schwartz RH, Hawks RL. Laboratory detection of marijuana use. *JAMA.* 254(6):788–792, 1985.
15. Mitchell J. Chemical balance. *Employee Assist.* October 1989; 2(3):12–17ff.

9

Eating Disorders
and Substance Abuse

Recently, there has been a growing awareness of the
relationship between eating disorders and substance
abuse. This area is of interest to clinicians not only for
their involvement in the etiology of cocaine abuse but
also for the challenges it presents in the successful diagnosis and treatment of addiction. The well-known
denial associated with use of a single drug may be
complicated by the patient's reluctance to admit an
eating disorder, as well as the reluctance of patients
with eating disorders to admit to drug use. This reluctance may stem from ignorance (for example, patients
may not realize how their eating disorder affects their
cocaine consumption). Or the patient—having one
form of substance abuse detected—may "sacrifice" this
substance so that other forms of substance abuse or
eating disorder can continue. Furthermore, clinicians,

having identified one abused substance, may not press to uncover other abused substances. These clinicians may believe that correcting one problem is difficult enough without the added burden of another. As a result, the association between eating disorders and substance abuse, specifically cocaine, deserves greater attention.

The Demographics of Eating Disorders

By averaging published studies, the current rate of binge eating in women is estimated to be 35%, with an estimated 8% reporting self-induced vomiting and 5.8% laxative abuse.[1] Anorexia nervosa is thought to be less prevalent, occurring in approximately 0.5 to 1.0% of young women.[2] Although eating disorders can occur at any age, adolescence is the typical age of onset. Among men, the rate of eating disorders is significantly less (although the use of anabolic steroids by males to attain an idealized physique may be another form of eating disorder).

Both anorexia nervosa and bulimia share their primary symptom: the pursuit of an idealized body shape (thinness) through food deprivation, excessive exercising, and/or purging. The consequences of these conditions can be fatal: Mortality rates among anorexic patients may approach 22%.[3] The mortality and morbidity rates for bulimia have not been established; however, this condition is frequently associated with a variety of harmful conditions, including substance abuse.

The incidence of substance abuse in patients with eating disorders has been recognized for several years. In 1968, Crips noted that anorexic and bulimic patients "present with alcoholism."[4] Several surveys of patients with eating disorders have uncovered a high rate of drug abuse. Beary et al. reported that 50% of their bulimic patients had significant substance abuse problems,[5] and Cantwell et al. found that 23% of their anorexic patients suffered from alcohol abuse or alcoholism.[6] A recent study by Kendler et al. reported an alcoholism rate of 15.5% among 123 subjects with broadly defined bulimia.[7] They estimated that lifetime risk for DSM-III-R bulimia in women to be 4.2%, increasing to 8% if probable bulimia syndromes are included.

Similarly, studies of chemically dependent subjects have revealed a high rate of eating disorders. We reported interviews of 157 consecutive inpatient admissions to a psychiatric hospital.[8] Of the 21 cocaine abusers within this sample, 6 had a clinical diagnosis of either anorexia nervosa or bulimia, and all were correctly identified by clinicians and questionnaires.

Hudson et al. examined 386 consecutive inpatients admitted to the Alcohol and Drug Treatment Center at McLean Hospital and asked them to fill out a questionnaire designed to make current or past diagnoses of anorexia nervosa and bulimia nervosa.[9] Twenty-two (15%) of the 143 women had a lifetime diagnosis of an eating disorder, and 12 of 143 had a current diagnosis of an eating disorder. Among men only two (1%) had a lifetime diagnosis. The 22 women with a lifetime diagnosis of an eating disorder all abused either stimulants or alcohol, or both. The eating disorder preceded development of drug abuse by at least 1 year in 50% of cases and developed at least 1 year after the onset of drug abuse in 36%. Furthermore, this study indicated a preference for stimulants among patients with eating disorders: Women with eating disorders were more likely than women without eating disorders to use a stimulant drug and less likely than other women patients to use an opiate drug. Clearly, these studies indicated a strong relationship between eating disorders and substance abuse.

Theories behind the Comorbidity of Eating Disorders and Substance Abuse

Several hypotheses have been proposed to account for the association between eating disorders and substance abuse. One theory suggests that eating disorders and substance abuse may be manifestations of an underlying addiction or a psychiatric problem such as major depressive disorder. Observed behaviors directed at food by bulimics certainly resemble those observed with substance abusers. In addition, medications used in the experimental treatment of bulimia include naltrexone, antidepressants, and other medications used in the treatment of drug withdrawal and relapse prevention. This theory of a common underlying pathology is supported by the increased frequency of alcoholism and depression in the families of patients with eating disorders. One study of bulimics and their families found that 51% of the bulimics had at least one first-degree relative with substance abuse problems.[10]

Another theory suggests that patients with eating disorders use cocaine and other stimulants as a means of controlling their weight. Partly to test this hypothesis, we administered a structured diagnostic interview to 259 consecutive callers to the national cocaine "hotline" who met DSM-III-R criteria for cocaine abuse[11] (see Table 9.1). The interview assessed all DSM-III-R criteria for eating disorders, generated lifetime diagnoses of anorexia nervosa and bulimia, provided data on frequency and duration of bingeing and purging behavior, and supplied information about drug habits and the influence of drug use on eating patterns. Fifty-seven (22%) of the 259 cocaine abusers met DSM-III-R criteria for bulimia, and 9% of the sample had a lifetime diagnosis of anorexia nervosa (2% with anorexia nervosa alone and 7% with anorexia nervosa and bulimia). This rate of anorexia nervosa was much higher than the 0.5% to 3.0% lifetime prevalence rates reported in other studies. The fact that these individuals suffered from actual eating disorders is supported by a number of other findings. Cocaine abusers with an eating disorder were significantly more likely to seek psychiatric treatment for an eating disorder; were significantly more likely to use cathartics, diet pills, and diuretics for weight loss and as a means of purging; and were significantly more likely to experience cessation of their menses compared with cocaine abusers who had no diagnosed eating disorders.

Although this study supported the link between eating disorders and substance abuse, the theory that cocaine might "self-medicate" eating disorders was not supported. Only 26% of the bulimic group and 0% of the anorexia nervosa group stated that cocaine helped their eating disorder.

A third theory posits that dieting increases drug self-administration. Food deprivation has been shown to increase the preferences for sweet foods in humans and for a wide variety of abused drugs, including alcohol, cocaine, amphetamine, heroin, and nicotine, in

TABLE 9.1. Diagnostic Characteristics of 259 Cocaine Abusers

Diagnosis

	Anorexia nervosa (N = 6)		Bulimia (N = 57)		Both (N = 19)		Bulimia[a] with purging (N = 24)		Bulimia without purging (N = 52)		No eating disorder (N = 177)	
	N	%	N	%	N	%	N	%	N	%	N	%
Male	1	17	25	44	1	5	6	25	20	38	95	54
Female	5	83	32	56	18	95	18	75	32	62	82	46
Menses stopped	3	60	9	28	12	67	11	61	10	31	12	15
History of binge eating	2	33	57	100	19	100	24	100	52	100	54	31
Self-induced vomiting	0	—	12	21	12	63	24	100	0	—	1	1
Psychiatric treatment for binge eating or weight loss	2	33	7	12	7	37	7	29	7	13	5	3
Drug-related eating symptoms	2	33	27	47	6	32	9	38	24	46	66	37
Drugs help eating symptoms	0	—	15	26	3	16	3	13	15	29	8	5
Diet pill abuse	2	33	32	56	14	74	16	67	30	58	32	18
Laxative abuse	1	17	6	11	3	16	5	21	4	8	7	4
Diuretic abuse	0	—	10	18	8	42	8	33	10	19	8	5

[a]Groupings for bulimia with purging and bulimia without purging were obtained from the entire sample of bulimic subjects (i.e., obtained from subjects with bulimia alone and with diagnoses of both anorexia nervosa and bulimia).

SOURCE: Jonas JM, Gold MS, Sweeney D, Pottash ALC. Eating disorders and cocaine abusers. *The Journal of Clinical Psychiatry* 48:47–50, 1987. Copyright 1987, Physicians Postgraduate Press. Reprinted with permission.

188

animals.[2] According to this theory, food deprivation alters the central reward mechanism and enhances the reinforcing effects of sweet foods and drugs of abuse. Supporting this theory is the fact that patients with eating disorders report greater pleasure from sweet substances than do controls.[12] Cocaine, already a potent reinforcer, may garner an even greater reinforcement effect in a food-deprived environment.

In addition, this theory would account for eating disorder onset preceding substance abuse. Jones et al. studied 27 cases where the eating disorder predated alcoholism.[13] Also, the 1948 study of normal men who had their calorie intake reduced by 50% found that coffee and tobacco consumption dramatically increased.[14]

A variation of this theory suggests that whenever one reinforcer is denied, other reinforcers increase. One study found that alcoholics who consumed the most sugar during the early stages of recovery had fewer relapses than the group that used less sugar.[15] This study confirms the common clinical observation of increased "junk food" and cigarette consumption in recovering alcoholics and drug addicts.[2]

Common Biological Pathways for Eating Disorders and Substance Abuse

An understanding of the neurochemistry of appetite suppression and cocaine's effect on appetite-regulating systems may explain at least partially the relationship between substance abuse and eating disorders.

The most important appetite-inhibiting neuropeptides include corticotropin releasing hormone, calcitonin gene-related peptide, neurotensin, and histididyl-prolinediketopiperazine, derived from TRH. Of specific interest is the relationship between neurotensin (NT) and dopamine (DA).

In the mesencephalon, NT-containing neurons originate in the ventral tegmental area (VTA) and terminate in the neighboring substantia nigra pars compacta (SNC), the nucleus accumbens (Acb), the caudate putamen, the prefrontal cortex (PFC), and the central median amygdala. In the diencephalon, NT is found within the zona incerta and the median eminence.

Both NT and dopamine are co-localized in neuronal projections from the VTA to the SNC and PFC and within the tuberoinfundibular dopamine system (TIDA), particularly the median eminence.[16]

The neurotensin connection is important because of the linkages between neurotensin and dopamine and the recent findings in cocaine administration and withdrawal. Pilotte et al.[17] showed that chronic treatment with cocaine and withdrawal from cocaine affected NT binding in the mesocortical regions differently than it affected other areas. Within the mesocorticolimbic system, NT binding in the parabrachial pigmented nucleus of the ventral tegmental area was 67% lower in cocaine-treated rats immediately after or 10 days after their final cocaine administration. More NT binding was found in postsynaptic terminal areas of the VTA (prefrontal cortex, substantia nigra) 10 days after withdrawal from cocaine. NT binding in the nucleus accumbens was unaffected by cocaine or its withdrawal. Cocaine decreased NT binding in nonmesocorticolimbic areas, including the dorsal hypothalamic area and the zona incerta, but binding returned to normal 10 days after withdrawal from cocaine. The most striking effects occurred in the lateral prefrontal cortex, where NT binding increased threefold.

The most persistent alterations in NT binding after cocaine occurred in the VTA, in its long mesocortical projection to the PFC, and in its short intramesencephalic projection to the SNC. Repeated microinjection of NT into the VTA increases locomotor activity and sensitization to subsequent injections of NT effects analogous to the behavioral sensitization seen with cocaine and amphetamine. Application of NT into the Acb attenuates the behavioral effects of amphetamine or stimulation of the VTA. The perikarya of DA-containing neurons within the SNC and the VTA bear NT binding sites, implying that NT can modulate these DA neurons. Direct application of NT into the VTA depolarizes the mesocorticolimbic DA neurons and liberates DA from terminals in the Acb. In this manner, NT acts much like cocaine, amphetamine, and other drugs of abuse.

Chronic cocaine administration and its withdrawal appear to disrupt the normal NT-DA interaction at both the cell bodies and the terminals. Cocaine-induced increase in NT binding in the PFC and the SNC may reflect a selective depletion of peptide from NT-DA neurons as a result of up-regulation of postsynaptic NT sites. This is analogous to the enhancement of DA binding. Because released peptides are not conserved through uptake as are monoamines, NT would be lost more readily than DA in the PFC. Thus chronic administration of cocaine may selectively deplete NT from VTA projections to the PFC and SNC without markedly affecting concentrations of DA or the reinforcing effects associated with enhanced DA levels.

The mesocortical and mesolimbic DA neurons have been implicated as essential in drug self-administration behavior maintained by cocaine. Pharmacological manipulations or lesions of the mesotelencephalic DA system significantly change place conditioning of abused substances, and this DA system apparently serves as an essential component for the central encoding in the brain of hedonic value associated with abusable compounds. In this manner, addictive drugs act on the reinforcing functions of the central nervous system in a manner analogous to biologically essential behaviors such as eating and sex. The abusive behaviors of food associated with eating disorders—repeated episodes of bingeing and starvation—apparently mimic the cocaine addict's common pattern of intermittent bingeing followed by periods of abstinence.

Treatment Implications

Perhaps the greatest problem associated with treating substance abuse complicated by eating disorders stems from a lack of familiarity with the optimum treatment strategies for each condition. Often, a clinician or treatment program experienced with the treatment of one of the conditions may simply attempt to transpose strategies effective for one discipline onto the other. At first this may seem understandable, since treatment strategies for both conditions share similar elements. For example, management of severe physical sequelae through either detoxification (for drugs) or nutritional supplement (for eating disorders) may be the first stage of treatment for either condition. Both conditions also require confrontation of the patient's denial combined with the application of appropriate educational efforts. Later, similar cognitive and behavioral strategies may be applied to help patients in their recovery.

However, patients suffering from an eating disorder may have difficulty accepting strategies commonly applied in the treatment of substance abuse. For example, a key tenet in a substance abuse program may involve helping patients to understand their powerlessness over the abused substance (the first step in AA). Conversely, patients with eating disorders often struggle with issues of control (many feel helpless and attempt to exert control over their food intake) and may react with extreme negativism if their attempts at control are threatened.[18] Similarly, the development of an eating disorder will usually predate the substance problem and often involves complicated family relationships, emotional problems, and feelings of worthlessness that may require specific psychotherapy. Also, positive societal attitudes regarding thinness compared to the negative views that surround drug abuse make the rewards of stopping the eating disorder behavior not as immediately apparent to the patient as the rewards that may follow substance abuse cessation. For example, employers may wholeheartedly support substance abuse treatment, but their support for eating disorder treatment may not be as strong. Finally, it is obviously impossible for a patient with an eating disorder to practice the total abstinence that most substance abuse treatment programs require. Therefore, an effective treatment program should treat these conditions concomitantly and with sensitivity to the needs of each disorder.

References

1. Fairburn CG, Beglin SJ. Studies of the epidemiology of bulimia nervosa. *Am J Psychiatry.* 1990;147:401–408.
2. Krahn DD. The relationship of eating disorders and substance abuse. *J Substance Abuse.* 1991;3:239–253.
3. Mitchell JE. *Anorexia Nervosa and Bulimia: Diagnosis and Treatment.* Minneapolis: University of Minnesota Press; 1985.
4. Crisp AH. Primary anorexia nervosa. *Gut.* 1968;9:370–372.
5. Beary MD, Lacey JH, Merry J. Alcoholism and eating disorders in women of fertile age. *Br J Addiction.* 1986;81:685–689.
6. Cantwell DP, Sturzenberg S, Burrough J, et al. Anorexia nervosa: an affective disorder? *Arch Gen Psychiatry.* 1977;34:1087–1093.
7. Kendler KS, MacLean C, Neale M, et al. The genetic epidemiology of bulima nervosa. *Am J Psychiatry.* 1991;148:1627–1637.
8. Jonas JM, Gold MS. Cocaine abuse and eating disorders. *Lancet.* 1(8477):390, 1986.
9. Hudson JI, Weiss RD, Pope HG Jr, et al. Eating disorders in hospitalized substance abusers. *Am J Drug Alcohol Abuse.* 1992; 18(1):75–85.
10. Carroll K, Leon G. The bulimic-vomiting disorder within a generalized substance abuse pattern. Paper presented at the Association for the Advancement of Behavior Therapy Annual Meeting, Toronto; 1981.
11. Jonas JM, Gold MS, Sweeney D, Pottash ALC. Eating disorders and cocaine abuse: a survey of 259 cocaine abusers. *J Clin Psychiatry.* 1987;48:47–50.
12. Drewenowski A, Halmi KA, Pierce B, et al. Taste and eating disorders. *Am J Nutrition.* 1987;46:442–450.
13. Jones DA, Cheshire N, Morehouse H. Anorexia nervosa, bulimia, and alcoholism—association of eating disorder and alcohol. *J. Psychiatric Res.* 1985;19:377–380.
14. Franklin JC, Schiele BC, Brozek J, Keys A. Observations on human behavior in experimental semistarvation and rehabilitation. *J Clin Psychol.* 1948;4:28–45.
15. Yung L, Gordis E, Holt J. Dietary choices and likelihood of abstinence among alcoholic patients in an outpatient clinic. *Drug Alcohol Depend.* 1983;12:355–362.
16. Kasckow J, Nemeroff CB. The neurobiology of neurotensin:

focus on neurotensin–dopamine interactions. *Regulatory Peptides.* 1991;26:153–164.

17. Pilotte NS, Mitchell WM, Sharpe LG, et al. Chronic cocaine administration and withdrawal of cocaine modify neurotensin binding in rat brain. *Synapse.* 1991;9:111–120.
18. Zweben JE. Eating disorders and substance abuse. *J Psychoactive Drugs.* 1987;19(2):181–192.

10

Physicians, the Elderly, Adolescents, and Substance Abuse

In any discussion of substance abuse there is a tendency to view patients as a homogeneous entity presenting with similar symptoms and responding alike to treatment. Rarely is the clinician so lucky. Specific subgroups have been discussed throughout this text, and this chapter focuses on many of these groups in greater detail.

The Medical Profession

In a book written primarily for clinicians, perhaps no special group is more important than the medical profession itself. Drug use among medical professionals is not a new phenomenon: At the turn of this century, one-third of the cocaine and opiate addicts were health care professionals.[1] Identifying physician addiction is complicated by the physicians' ability to rationalize their drug use and avoid detection, factors that contribute to the wall of denial surrounding the addicted physician.

Drug Use among Medical Students and Residents

Although the exact rate of drug abuse among all physicians is not known, a study of medical residents found past-year and past-month use of cocaine to be 6.1% and 1.8%, respectively.[2] Among medical students, rates of cocaine abuse were higher: Past-year and past-month use of cocaine were 10.1% and 2.8%, respectively.[3] These self-reported rates for both residents and medical students were less than their age-matched cohorts (who may be less afraid of being honest), but an alarming 20% of the residents indicated that they knew other physicians they considered to be impaired by drug and alcohol abuse.[4]

Although impaired physicians frequently identify medical school as the period most critical to the development of their impairment, their drug use usually predates medical school admission. In one study of alcohol-abusing medical students, 63% had a history of abuse prior to medical school.[5] Similarly, the 1987 study of medical students reported that of the medical students using cocaine, 72.6% began their cocaine use in college (compared to 13.2% who began in medical school).[3] Nevertheless, the stress of medical school and the lack of social support, combined with the neglect by many medical schools to emphasize anti-drug efforts, have contributed to a fertile drug-using environment. Figure 10.1 illustrates past year substance abuse by specialty of medical residents.

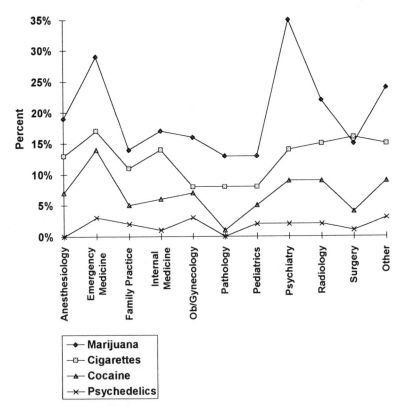

FIGURE 10.1. Past year substance abuse by medical residents. SOURCE: Hughes, PH, Conrad, SE, Baldwin, DC, et al. Resident physician substance abuse in the United States. *JAMA.* 1991; 265(16); 2069-2073.

Another study of medical, nursing, premedical, and young physicians found a lifetime rate of marijuana use ranging from 56 to 70%, with 15 to 21% of these users progressing to other illegal drugs (including cocaine).[6] Drug use by medical students may go undetected because medical schools do not routinely screen for drug use and because many medical students and residents may hesitate to report their drug use for fear of ruining their chances at a successful medical career. Also, residents often report that they take drugs and alcohol as a means to survive the rigors of medical training; when the drugs "work," they're taken again. Having established that they "can get away with drug use" while surviving medical training makes these physicians candidates for addiction.

Furthermore, Clark et al. reported that young residents develop poor prescribing habits.[7] Having recently gained the power to prescribe medication, these residents often dole out prescriptions indiscriminately to themselves and/or to friends and relatives seeking free medical advice and treatment. Table 10.1 details the liberality of resident prescribing practices—practices that may portend future substance abuse problems.

Drug Use among Physicians

Several factors besides exposure during medical school and residency contribute to physician drug abuse.

First, there is *access*. Doctors have relatively easy access to a wide range of potentially addicting medications. Physicians have been known to "eat the mail" (consuming free samples of medications) and to self-prescribe medications for dubious reasons.

Second, there is *familiarity*. Many physicians prescribe powerful and potentially addicting medications on a daily, even hourly, basis. Over time, this close association often dulls a physician's wariness regarding these medications.

Third, there is a *false security*. With a detailed

TABLE 10.1. Resident Physician Substance Abuse

Substance	N	Self-treament	Under physician's supervision	Performance/wakefulness	Recreational	Dependent on it	Other reasons
Amphetamines	42	16.7	0	76.2	23.0	2.4	9.5
Barbituates	28	46.4	35.7	7.1	39.3	0	7.1
Benzodiazepines	188	75.0	15.4	2.7	6.9	0	14.4
Opiates	62	51.6	35.5	3.2	27.4	0	6.5

SOURCE: Hughes PH, Conrad SE, Baldwin DC, et al. Resident physician substance abuse in the United States. *JAMA.* 1991; 265(16);2069–2073. Copyright 1991, American Medical Association. Reprinted with permission.

knowledge of human anatomy and physiology, many physicians assume that this knowledge gives them power over a drug, whether it be a prescription medication or an illicit drug. They assume that they will be able to control a drug and stop before addiction occurs, since they think they know how a drug works as well as the signs of addiction. This assumption is just another example of how denial can help drug users rationalize their drug taking. And addicted physicians often see their failure to control their addiction as a professional failing, even shame, which may prevent them from seeking treatment.

Fourth, there is *ignorance*. Medical education of physicians has often neglected the study of substance abuse in general and impaired physicians in particular. By not giving these problems adequate attention, medical schools have contributed to substance abuse in our society and in their profession.

Fifth, there is *attitude*. When compared to high school students, medical students are more likely to accept the occasional or experimental use of cocaine. In the survey of medical students, 20.6% would take no action in response to the occasional use of cocaine;[3] however, 93.9% of high school seniors disapproved of adults using cocaine even once or twice.[8]

Characteristics of the Impaired Physician

A study of impaired physicians found that the majority abused alcohol.[9] However, the study found that the incidence of cocaine and parenteral drug abuse appeared to be rising in the late 1980s. Over 96% of the physicians in this study were male, while the national percentage of male physicians at that time was 86%. The authors noted that anesthesiologists and general practitioners were overrepresented. Older physicians tended to abuse a single drug (usually alcohol), whereas younger physicians were more likely to abuse multiple drugs. Other studies have found a greater tendency for poly-drug abuse among pharmacists and nurses.[10]

Substance abuse appears to be a significant factor in physician suicide. In fact, one study found that substance abuse was the greatest difference between deceased by suicide physicians and deceased nonsuicide physicians: 34% of the deceased by suicide group had a history of substance abuse compared to 14% of the deceased non-suicide physicians.[11] Among the suicide physicians, more than 50% had self-prescribed a psychoactive medication, compared to only 22% of the nonsuicide group.

Identifying the Impaired Physician

The following signs are some of the major indications of an impaired physician.[12]

- Disruptions in family life*
- Legal problems
- Neglectful of practice routines
- Social isolation
- Driving while intoxicated
- Noticeable odor of alcohol at the work site
- Making hospital rounds at unusual hours

---

*Reprinted from Harris, BA. Not enough is enough. The physician who is dependent on alcohol and other drugs. *N.Y.S. J. Med* 86(1):2–3, 1986. Copyright by the Medical Society of the State of New York and reprinted with permission.

- Canceling office appointments without obvious conflicts of time
- Giving unusual or dangerous orders over the telephone, particularly from home during the evening or night
- Disruptive behavior at meetings, or failure to complete committee assignments
- Forgetting social appointments
- Holding telephone conversations with slurred speech or tangential conversations
- Dressing sloppily or in a noticeably different style

The above signs are primarily based on the abuse of alcohol, but physicians are also prone to abuse drugs through self-injection. Signs of self-injected drug abuse include septic, necrotic skin lesions and hardened, fibrositic changes of muscular tissue.[13]

Treating the Substance-Abusing Physician

The status afforded physicians, their position as authority figures, their training background that fosters self-reliance, and their emotional detachment and discipline are all factors that mitigate against the drug-abusing physician's acceptance of treatment. In addition there is still a lack of acceptance of the disease concept of addiction among many physicians, and this lack of acceptance may cause addicted physicians to stigmatize their addiction as a moral failure, thereby making the acceptance of treatment more difficult.

Fortunately, the American Medical Association and most state medical societies have addressed the problem of impaired physicians through specialized identification, education, and treatment programs. The success of employee assistance programs (EAPs) has stimulated the growth of peer assistance programs for physicians. Based on the EAP model, these programs use intervention, family therapy, and addiction-treatment programs geared for the physician. Given treatment, the outlook for the addicted physician is quite favorable. Two studies have found treatment success rates of 75 and 83% for impaired physicians.[13]

The Elderly and Substance Abuse

Although drug use is commonly seen as a problem of the young, elderly persons are at substantial risk for addiction given their frequent use of prescription medication. Although the elderly represent only 13% of the population, they take 25% of all prescription drugs and 70% of all nonprescription medications. It is not unusual for the typical elderly person to have one or more long-term illnesses, such as arthritis, heart disease, or diabetes. As a result, the elderly person may consume a bewildering amount of medications, prescribed by a multitude of physicians. Given this situation, the opportunity for serious drug interactions or medication mismanagement leading to prescription drug abuse is significant.

Although data concerning the use of illegal drugs by the elderly are lacking, we do know that 31 million Americans are over 65 years old, with an estimated 2 million alcoholics over the age of 60. Considering the fact that even low doses of cocaine can produce intercranial hemorrhage, cocaine use by this population poses special risks of cerebral vascular accidents.

As our population ages, we will undoubtedly see an increase in cocaine use by the elderly. In fact, the most recent NIDA survey did find an increase in monthly cocaine use among people over the age of 35 (see Chapter 1). Studies examining the best treatment modalities for this elderly population are necessary.

Adolescents and Substance Abuse

In 1991, an estimated 7.8% of the high school senior class of 1991 had used cocaine at least once.[14] Although this is a significant decline from the 17.3% of the high school seniors who had used cocaine in 1985, it nevertheless indicates that there is a significant percentage of adolescents willing to use cocaine.

More recent data from PRIDE indicates that drug use among students may be increasing.[15] PRIDE surveys of 212, 802 students during the 1991–1992 school year indicated that for junior high students (grades 6–8), drug use rose in all 10 categories (cigarettes, beer, wine coolers, liquor, marijuana, cocaine, uppers, downers, hallucinogens, and inhalants.) Among high school students, drug use rose in 7 of 10 categories, declining in only 3 drug types (wine coolers, marijuana, and cocaine). Perhaps PRIDE's most alarming finding concerns the dramatic increase in hallucinogen use: an 8% increase since 1990–1991 and a 20% increase since the 1988–1989 school year. (See pp. 218–219 for more information.)

Chapter 2 discusses how the Partnership for a Drug-Free America has used an effective media and educational campaign to "unsell" drugs to adolescents and adults alike. Unfortunately, other media and promotional advertising campaigns have had the effect of selling tobacco and alcohol to adolescents. Tobacco and alcohol are "gateway" drugs: One study found that more than half of the high school seniors who used cocaine began drinking beer and smoking cigarettes at age 13 or under; a third of them began their involvement with alcohol and tobacco before the age of 11.[1]

Alcohol use by young people has significant social consequences. According to US Surgeon General Novello, 52% of college students report using alcohol before committing crimes and 70% of attempted suicides involved frequent use of alcohol. Novello also reported alcohol use associated with over 27% of all murders, 30% of rapes, 33% of all property offenses, and 37% of robberies by young people.

Promoting Cigarettes to Adolescents

A recent study examined the effectiveness of a major advertising campaign in promoting cigarettes to adolescents and adults.[16] The study used four standard marketing measures (recognition, recall, appeal, and brand preference) in comparing the adolescent and adult responses to a specific advertising campaign—RJR Nabisco's "Old Joe" cartoon character campaign for Camel cigarettes. A total of 1055 high school students (mean age 15.99 years) and 345 adults aged 21 years or older (mean age 40.47 years) were surveyed.

The study found that the Old Joe Camel cartoon advertisements were far more successful at promoting Camel cigarettes to adolescents than to adults. For example, adolescents were more likely to:

- Recognize the cartoon character (97.7% of adolescents versus 72.2% of adults)

- Identify the product being advertised (97.5% of adolescents versus 67% of adults)
- Remember the Camel brand name (93.6% of adolescents versus 57.7% of adults)

The adolescents also found the cartoon campaign to be more appealing. Fifty-eight percent of the adolescents thought the Old Joe character was "cool" (compared to 39.9% of the adults), while 73.6% of the adolescents thought he was "interesting" (versus 55.1% of the adults).

Advertising campaigns similar to Camel's may explain why cigarettes are so popular among young smokers. The 1991 National High School Senior Survey found that 44% of eighth graders had already tried cigarettes, with 14% having smoked at least one cigarette within the last 30 days.

Until the advent of the Old Joe campaign, Camel cigarettes were traditionally not popular with these young smokers. Surveys of smokers between the 7th and 12th grades, conducted between 1974 and 1988, found that only 0.5% preferred Camels. In 1986, Camels were most popular with smokers 65 years and older and least popular with 17- to 24-year-old smokers.[17]

However, in 1988, RJR Nabisco began the cartoon campaign with its Old Joe character reportedly based on a combination of James Bond and Don Johnson of "Miami Vice." DiFranza and colleagues suggest that tobacco marketeers use campaigns such as Camel's in an attempt to exploit the major psychological weaknesses of adolescents and children. One Camel advertisement depicts a cowboy being denied admission to a party because only "smooth characters" need apply (that is, Camel smokers). As a result, the researchers conclude that "children use tobacco, quite simply, because they believe the benefits outweigh the risks. To the insecure child these benefits are the 'psychological benefits' promised in tobacco advertisements: confidence, an improved image, and popularity."[16]

Since the debut of the Old Joe campaign, Camel's popularity with young smokers has soared. By 1991, brand preference for Camel among smokers under the age of 18 improved from 0.5 to 32.8%. The researchers estimated that the revenues from the illegal sale of Camel cigarettes to children grew from $6 million per year in 1987 to $476 million per year in 1991.

The authors conclude their study by stating, "Our study provides further evidence that tobacco advertising promotes and maintains nicotine addiction among children and adolescents. A total ban of tobacco advertising and promotions, as part of an effort to protect children from the dangers of tobacco, can be based on sound scientific reasoning."[16]

Because a total ban on cigarette advertising and promotions is unlikely in the very near future, physicians must stress the importance of eliminating all forms of substance abuse in adolescents. Physicians should ask specific questions, intervene with the child, and appeal to parents and family members—not only to inform them about the dangers of adolescent substance abuse but also to provide them with effective antidrug strategies.

Family Strategies in Adolescent Drug Abuse

The following list presents suggestions that physicians can use to help parents prevent drug use by their children.

- Encourage parents to continue their drug education by reading more and talking with other parents and school officials. Getting involved with school and local drug programs will help to keep them aware of developments in your community. The drug abuse picture in this country changes frequently, as new drugs and new methods of abuse emerge with alarming regularity.
- Stress to parents the importance of realizing how parental attitudes about drugs—not just illicit drugs but also alcohol, cigarettes, and even caffeine and prescription medications—can influence their offspring. In a 1990 study conducted by the Partnership for a Drug-Free America, 26% of all teens surveyed reported that their parents have used marijuana, 8% say their parents have used cocaine, and 3% say their parents have used crack.[18] Fourteen percent of the teens surveyed say they have wished that their parent or someone else living in their home would stop using illegal drugs. The researchers concluded that "family drug use is directly related to teens' own use of drugs. The incidence of drug use among children of parents who have tried drugs is much higher than among children who report that their parents have not tried drugs."
- Help parents to understand that adolescent attitudes can be used to prevent drug abuse. For example:
  - Almost half of the teenagers who use marijuana regularly fear that they will get caught by the law. An even greater

number fear getting caught by parents or school authorities.

o Roughly 4 out of 10 adolescents fear that their own drug use will negatively influence their brothers or sisters.

o One teenager in three is afraid of getting hold of impure marijuana; twice that number fear impure cocaine or crack.

o Nearly 6 out of 10 teenagers fear that cocaine use will lead to physical or psychological damage; half of them fear becoming dependent on the drug.[19]

Parents can use these fearful attitudes in constructive ways by teaching their children that there is good reason not to start using drugs now, or to stop now if currently using drugs.

• Inform parents of the risk factors for drug abuse as well as the signs of abuse (see Table 10.2). Stress that after parental and sibling drug use, the next area of concern is drug use by the child's friends.

TABLE 10.2. Risk Factors for Adolescent Drug Abuse

Parental alcohol or drug problems
Use of drugs by siblings
Peer involvement with drugs
Poor parent-child communication
Access to illegal drugs
Divorce, financial difficulties, or other sources of family stress
A preexisting psychological or behavioral problem

SOURCE: Adapted with permission from Gold MS. *The Good News About Drugs and Alcohol.* New York: Villard Books, 1991:178.

- Emphasize the importance of early intervention. For the safety of children, intervention *must* take place if their relationship to drugs has grown stronger than any other relationship in their life. Intervention may take several forms: from searching a child's room, to doing annual urine screens during pediatric checkups, to seeking professional help. Some parents feel hesitant to invoke any of these interventions, especially searching children's rooms. However, parents who suspect their child of using drugs have a right—even an obligation—to intervene. Any room, including a child's bedroom, is a part of the parent's home, and no activity that threatens the health of a child should ever be permitted.

Treating the Adolescent Cocaine User

The treatment of adolescent substance abusers requires many special considerations. First, the physician should not automatically assume that a dysfunctional family contributed to the adolescent's substance abuse. Even a dysfunctional family is present at the time of treatment; their dysfunction may have resulted from the adolescent's substance abuse.

The clinician should also be aware that the adolescent patient may not be able to understand intellectually or emotionally many of the tenets of treatment programs. Specifically, many of the treatment strategies that work for adults, such as the Twelve Steps of AA, may not be as effective in adolescent populations. The complexity of many of the Twelve Steps, such as Step

4, "Made a searching and fearless moral inventory of ourselves," and Step 10, "Continued to take a personal inventory and when we were wrong promptly admitted it," often requires that the Twelve Steps be presented and explained as clearly as possible to the adolescent patient.

Even the first step ("We admitted that we were powerless over alcohol—that our lives had become unmanageable") may be especially difficult for an adolescent to embrace. Many adolescents already feel powerless over their lives, and the fact that most of the adolescents are coerced to enter treatment only adds to the feeling of powerlessness. Adolescents may find it especially difficult to relinquish what they perceive to be their only power: their "control" over their drug consumption. Anger at their feelings of powerlessness may translate into acting out behavior during the early stages of treatment.

Furthermore, many of the goals of adult treatment, such as a return to work, simply do not apply for the adolescent user. Instead, adolescent therapy should therefore stress the possibility and importance of socialization in a nondrug environment.[20] Participation in age-appropriate group therapy or AA groups for adolescents helps to reinforce the benefits of socializing with nondrug users.

Clinicians should also realize that the young cocaine user frequently abuses other substances. In Chapter 4, the medical complications of multiple drugs of abuse were discussed. The following section explores some of the treatment challenges posed by the abuse of multiple substances.

Multiple Substances of Abuse

Among cocaine abusers who abuse other drugs, alcohol is the most likely substance to be abused. In treatment populations of adults and adolescents, between 70 and 90% of cocaine addicts are alcoholics.[21] The Epidemiologic Catchment Area Study of the general population found an 84% alcoholism rate among cocaine addicts (see Figure 10.2).[22]

The physician may have to probe deeply to uncover the alcohol abuse. Cocaine users may deny that they do not use alcohol or derive any effects from its use. They may not even be aware of the extent of their alcohol abuse or may label it as normal, since many alcoholic abusers have distorted perceptions of what normal drinking is.[23] They may mistakenly believe that all drinkers drink to get inebriated or to solve personal

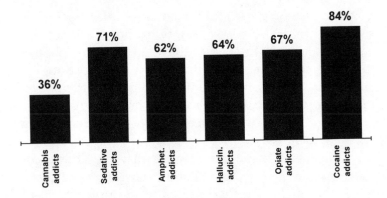

FIGURE 10.2. Prevalence of alcoholism among other drug users. SOURCE: Robins, LN, et al. Alcohol disorders in the community: A report from the Epidemiologic Catchment Area. In Rose, RM, Barret, J (eds.). *Alcoholism: Origins and Outcome.* New York: Raven Press, 1988.

or emotional problems. Frequently, they think that the only difference between themselves and normal drinkers is the fact that "the normal drinkers haven't been caught yet."

The high frequency of multiple drug use by cocaine users argues favorably for the widespread use of urine screens as a diagnostic and treatment aid. Similarly, the vulnerability of cocaine users to other drugs of abuse supports a basic tenet of most treatment programs: the complete avoidance of all mood-altering substances during recovery.

Alcohol is the most common concomitant drug of abuse, but other drugs less familiar to the clinician may also be abused by cocaine addicts. Two of these drugs that have recently garnered attention are "Ecstasy" and "Ice."

Ecstasy

Ecstasy belongs to the family of drugs known as methoxylated amphetamines—essentially a cross between a stimulant and a hallucinogen. Ecstasy is actually methylenedioxymethamphetamine, or MDMA, but similar compounds, such as MDA and MMDA, are also sold under the same name. MDMA was first synthesized in 1914, but its use didn't begin to gain popularity until the late 1970s.

Ecstasy's alleged ability to facilitate interpersonal communication and intimacy led to its experimental use as an adjunct to psychotherapy. Much like the early claims that surrounded cocaine's introduction in the 1880s, the early ancedotal reports about Ecstasy led to the mistaken impression that it was both psychologically beneficial and physically harmless. Media reports in the 1980s helped to popularize Ecstasy as the "love drug" or "hug drug." Therapists believed that patients who used this drug would be more open and honest with each other. But the therapeutic value of the drug has never been proved. The drug's surge in popularity, combined with reports of adverse side effects, led the Drug Enforcement Administration to classify MDMA as a Schedule One drug, thereby banning its manufacture, sale, possession, or use.

A recent study of 100 Ecstasy users in Sydney, Australia, found that users experienced a "positive mood state" 94% of the time when taking the drug. However, "unpleasant side effects" were reported 86% of the time Ecstasy was used. In this study, 77% of the Ecstasy users had tried cocaine, with 26% stating that they currently use cocaine.[23]

The overall number of positive reactions to Ecstasy led the Sydney researchers to ask, "Given that Ecstasy has so many positive aspects, why isn't it being used more often?" The results of their survey helped to answer this question: Users reported that the pleasurable effects decreased while negative side effects increased with repeated administration of the drug and/or high doses. Apparently, the fact that the unpleasant side effects quickly outweigh the pleasurable effects significantly limits the drug's use.

The negative side effects of Ecstasy are not surprising given the sympathomimetic nature of the drug. In the Sydney study, users reported adverse reactions such as fainting, decreased respiration, teeth grinding, paranoia, panic, loss of control, anxiety, hallucinations, nausea, and vomiting.

Furthermore, there is a growing body of evidence suggesting that MDMA has a neurotoxic effect on serotonergic nerve terminals.[25] A single large dose of MDMA given orally to monkeys has been found to deplete serotonin production in the thalamus and hypothalamus 2 weeks later.[26] The exact meaning these animal studies have for humans cannot be determined; nevertheless, they suggest that Ecstasy is not a drug to be taken lightly.

Methamphetamine ("Ice")

Ice is a form of crystallized methamphetamine that resembles chips of ice. Although Ice is a relative newcomer, methamphetamine was first synthesized in 1893 by a Japanese chemist. During World War II, the Japanese government attempted to improve productivity by giving methamphetamine to its soldiers and munitions workers. Use of the drug continued after the war, and as a result, Japan is currently the largest consumer market for methamphetamine.[27]

In 1986, methamphetamine in the form of Ice began to spread from the Far East into Hawaii. From there, the drug eventually migrated to the West Coast.

Ice and crack are similar in many ways: Both are smoked, both produce euphoria within seconds, both can cause serious physical and psychological side effects, and both can lead to violence. Police in Honolulu estimate that Ice may be involved in approximately 70% of their spouse-abuse cases.[28]

There is one major difference between the two: Whereas crack euphoria usually wears off in 15 minutes or less, the euphoria from Ice may last up to 24 hours. It is the length of the euphoria, combined with the powerful effects of methamphetamine, that has some drug treatment specialists worried. Ironically, the length of the euphoria may actually limit the drug's popularity, since it may make the drug less reinforcing (hence less addicting) than cocaine. Currently, the use of Ice appears to be limited to the West Coast.

The Resurgence of LSD: New Strategies Are Needed

PRIDE's recent survey of students demonstrated that hallucinogen use is increasing while cocaine use is decreasing (see Figure 10.3). Other independent data support our findings: While cocaine emergency room (ER) visits decreased between 1985 and 1990, LSD ER visits increased by 65%, according to the Drug Enforcement Administration (DEA). Half of the LSD ER visits nationwide are for children aged 10–19. In 1990 LSD seizures were the third largest of all dangerous drugs seized, according to the National Narcotics Intelligence Consumers Committee's June 1991 report. Five hun-

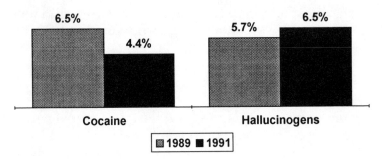

FIGURE 10.3. USA trends in teen drug use, 1989–1991. SOURCE: PRIDE, 1992.

dred thousand LSD dosage units were confiscated in the United States by the DEA in 1990. In addition, marijuana-use rates have steadily declined while the THC concentration and toxicity have increased. From the 1960s to the 1990s, THC potency has increased by 160% while LSD potency decreased by 560%. Analysis of seized LSD has consistently demonstrated that LSD has been reformulated in a lower dose (20–80mcg per unit dose versus 150–300mcg in the 1960s). But "low" dose LSD is not safe LSD. PRIDE interviews with high school students suggest that this reformulation has helped LSD overcome its "bad trips with flashbacks" image. Our most recent work indicates that many young people now believe that cocaine is dangerous but that LSD is spiritually uplifting, possibly providing a "therapeutic" or "religious" experience.

Perceptions of danger are important factors in the willingness to try an illicit drug. Today, more than 55% of high school seniors believe that trying LSD a few times is not harmful. Changes in unit dose and attitude may be contributing to the LSD resurgence: 1992 PRIDE surveys indicate a 20% increase in hallucinogen use by students since 1988 (Figure 10.3). Lessons from the recent cocaine epidemic have been overly specific and applied to cocaine alone. National prevention and educational efforts may need to be refocused, less drug-specific, and more consistent with the concept of the drug-free, healthy mind.

References

1. Gold MS. *The Good News About Drugs and Alcohol*. New York: Villard Books; 1991.

2. Hughes PH, Conrad SE, Baldwin DC, et al. Resident physician substance abuse in the United States. *JAMA.* 1991;265(16);2069–2073.

3. Baldwin DC, Hughes PH, Conrad SE, et al. Substance abuse among senior medical students. *JAMA.* 1991;265(16):2074–2078.

4. Conrad SE, Hughes P, Baldwin D, et al. Substance abuse and the resident physician: a national study. *Ann Conf Resident Med Ed.* 1988;27:256–261.

5. Clark DC. Alcohol and drug use and mood disorders among medical students: implications for physician impairment. *Q.R.B.* 1988;14(2):50–54.

6. McAuliffe WE, Rohman M, Fishman P, et al. Psychoactive drug use by young and future physicians. *J Health Soc Behav.* 1984;25:34–54.

7. Clark A, Kay J, Clark D. Patterns of psychoactive drug prescriptions by house officers for non-patients. *J Med Educ.* 1988; 63:44–50.

8. National Institute on Drug Abuse. 1991 Survey of High School Seniors; February 1992.

9. Talbot GD, Gallegos KV, Wilson PO, Porter TL. The Medical Association of Georgia's Impaired Physician Program. Review of the first 1000 physicians: analysis of specialty, *JAMA.* 1987;257(2):2927–2930.

10. Gallegos KV, Veit FW, Wilson PO, et al. Substance abuse among health professionals. *Md Med J.* 1988;37(3):191–197.

11. Council on Scientific Affairs. Results and implications of the AMA-APA physician mortality project, stage II. *JAMA.* 1987; 257(21):2949–2953.

12. Harris BA. Not enough is enough. The physician who is dependent on alcohol and other drugs. *N.Y.S. J Med.* 1986;86(1):2–3.

13. Collins GB. Drug and alcohol use and addiction among physicians. In: Miller NS, ed. *Comprehensive Handbook of Drug Addiction.* New York: Marcel Dekker; 1991: chap 52.

14. NIDA High School Senior Survey; February 1992.

15. High School Student Drug Use Rose in '91 for Most Drugs; In Junior High Usage Climbed in All Drug Types. PRIDE Press releases, October 19, 1992.

16. DiFranza JR, Richards JW, Paulman PM, et al. RJR Nabisco's

cartoon camel promotes Camel cigarettes to children. *JAMA.* 1991;266:3149–3153.

17. Centers for Disease Control. Cigarette brand use among adult smokers—United States, 1986. *MMWR.* 1990;39:665–673.
18. The Partnership Attitude Tracking Study: A Summary of the Fourth Year Results. The Gordon S. Black Corporation. The Partnership for a Drug-Free America; 1990.
19. Black GS. Changing attitudes toward drug use—1988. Reports from the Media-Advertising Partnership for a Drug-Free America, Inc. The Gordon S. Black Corporation.
20. Morehouse ER. Treating adolescent cocaine abusers. In: Washton AM, Gold MS, eds. *Cocaine: A Clinician's Handbook.* New York: The Guilford Press; 1987.
21. Miller NS, Gold MS. Comorbidity of drug and alcohol addictions: epidemiologial, familial and genetic evidence for common transmission. In press.
22. Helzer J, Burnam A. Epidemiology of alcohol addiction: United States. In: Miller NS, ed. *Comprehensive Handbook of Drug Addiction.* New York: Marcel Dekker; 1991.
23. Blume SB. Alcohol problems in cocaine abusers, In: Washton AM, Gold MS, eds. *Cocaine: A Clinician's Handbook.* New York: The Guilford Press; 1987.
24. Solowij N, Hall W, Lee N. Recreational MDMA use in Sydney: a profile of "ecstasy" users and their experiences with the drug. *Br J Addiction.* In press.
25. O'Hearn E, Battaglia G, DeSouza EB, et al. Methylenedioxyamphetamine (MDA) and methylenedioxymethamphetamine (MDMA) cause selective ablation of serotonergic axon terminals in the forebrain: immunocytochemical evidence for neurotoxicity. *J Neurosci.* 1988;8(8):2788–2803.
26. Ricaurte GA, Delanney LE, Irwin I, Langston JW. Toxic effects of MDMA on central serotonergic neurons in the primate: importance of route and frequency of drug administration. *Brain Res.* 1988;446:165–168.
27. National Council of Alcoholism and Drug Dependence, Inc. *10 Answers to Your Questions about "Ice."* New York; 1990.
28. U.S. Department of Justice. A special report on Ice. U.S. Department of Justice, Drug Enforcement Administration, Office of Intelligence; October 1989.

Index

223